# Think Yourself Free!

White Dog Seminars

PO Box 101
Darnum
3822 Victoria
Australia

National Library of Australia
Cataloguing-in-Publication data

Christopher Roering
**Think Yourself Free!**

ISBN 978-0-646-85507-3

Cover design and typesetting by Jethro Harcourt
Printed by IngramSpark

Published by White Dog Seminars, ABN 25 811 636 305
Correspondence to PO Box 101, Darnum, Victoria, Australia
christopherroering@dcsi.net.au

# Think Yourself Free!

How to change the way you think and act to overcome anxiety and depression and improve your mental health

**Christopher Roering**

# Acknowledgements

Thank you to my clients, over many years, who have been so courageous and ready for change. I have learnt from each one of you. You inspired and continue to inspire me! *This book represents my own opinions and is not intended to interfere with any medical or allied health treatments you might be having. It is intended to open the mind to new possibilities for natural treatment of anxiety and depression through changing the way we think and act.*

Thank you Tony Gilmour, author of the excellent book, *Tragic to Magic*, for your inspiration, and thank you to my editor, Alana Kiguchi Winfield. Thank you Captain Romeo Rusu for allowing me to write my book on the bridge of the giant container ship, *MV Guardian*. Thank you Jethro Harcourt for text and cover design. I am also grateful to my friends for their support: Uschi Goussard, Bev Lewis, Jane Pennells, Peter Savage, Bill and Kati Patterson, Jorge Robello and the Institute of Applied Psychology.

I dedicate this book to the memory of my wonderful parents and family.

I

# Foreword

*Foreword By Dr Bernadette Spencer. MBBS. RN1 Doctor at Monash Health and Teacher at the School of Health, Federation University.*

When dealing with mental health challenges, meaningful help is heartbreakingly difficult to access. Endless barriers exist to getting useful and timely assistance—so many hurdles that it becomes almost impossible for most people. Furthermore, the research into different therapies and techniques is diverse, endless, and extremely confusing. It is so easy to get lost in the sea of appointments, referrals, waiting lists, wellbeing exercises, medications, and advice. Becoming overwhelmed is almost inevitable, and this most often happens in times of crisis.

Fortunately for us as readers, Christopher has spent decades carefully combing through research, as well as contributing personally to it. He draws together techniques from many different disciplines and provides the reader with a simple, easy-to-read guide to improving many different aspects of the mind, relationships, and life.

He contrasts popular catchphrases against scientific evidence and offers a useful way for readers to navigate through both, to find true and meaningful help. He gives frequent, varied examples, and makes it clear that these tools can be applied to you and your life. You, as the reader, do not have to fit in to a certain box. You, as a person, are not broken, and it is not your fault.

This thought-provoking book is a breath of fresh air into the subject of contemporary mental health and happiness. Christopher provides simple, practical examples, explaining why common perceptions *are* common, and more importantly, he provides solutions. These tools can be used in the moment, then practised and learned. Eventually these thoughts and actions become automatic, with startling results.

This inspiring book is not only grounding and realistic in its recommendations but also conveys Christopher's kind and warm perspective. His sensible and sensitive nature shines through, as well as his quick wit. Reading this book provided me with the same sense of gentle encouragement, hope and optimism that I have always felt in my professional association with Chris, which is a true privilege. I am very grateful to Chris for his valuable contribution to mental health, and I am glad that through this book, he has made this opportunity available to you too.

# Contents

# Introduction

Over a decade ago, the World Health Organisation (WHO) declared mental illness to be the fourth most significant cause of suffering and disability worldwide (behind heart disease, cancer and traffic accidents) and predicted that it would rise to become the second most debilitating human condition by the year 2020. We reached that inglorious milestone in 2014! The WHO had to revise its forecasts — on 30 March 2017, the WHO declared mental disorders the leading cause of ill health and disability worldwide. Rates of depression worldwide have risen by more than 18% since 2005. The Director-General of the WHO at the time, Margaret Chan, said: 'These new figures are a wake-up call for all countries to rethink their approaches to mental health and to treat it with the urgency it deserves.' Currently one in four people in the world will be affected by mental disorders in their lifetime, and anxiety and depression are by far the most common mental disorders. We are more in debt, more obese, more addicted and more medicated, than we have ever been.

What does this mean for us? It tells us that anxiety and depression are pervasive and debilitating conditions, with high growth rates worldwide. It suggests that most of the people who need help don't receive it. Depression and anxiety will affect individuals, families and cultures in unpredictable ways and its growth is more likely to be socially transmitted than by other means. According to a research article by C. Davey and A. Chanen, published in the *Medical Journal of Australia*, May 2016, Australia has one of the highest rates of antidepressant use in the world. An article by Dr Martin Whitely published on 23 April 2019 in *Psychwatch Australia* states that 15% of Australians are taking antidepressant medication. In other words, one in eight Australians (over three million) are on antidepressants. The *Australian Institute of Health and Welfare* has revealed that more than 220,000 Australian children are medicated for mental illness. Data from the *Australian Institute of Health and Welfare* has shown that 2,312 toddlers and pre-school children were prescribed medication for mental illness from 2018–2019.

The Western World over recent decades has moved from 'can do' to 'can't do'. We are micromanaged by a bombardment from media, government, the bureaucracy and 'big business' about what we are not allowed to believe, what we are not allowed to do and what we are not allowed to say. Micromanagement is disempowering because it takes away choice and free thought and makes a major contribution to anxiety and depression. (Australia for instance is the only country in the world where we are not allowed to use our cell phones while refuelling our cars!)

Our flight response to this anxiety (manifesting in social withdrawal) can be seen in the fact that over 40% of Australians live on their own. (This includes single parents.) We are becoming more and more disconnected and isolated — exacerbated by the COVID challenge. Personal contact has dwindled since the advent of working from home, online meetings, online shopping, telehealth appointments, ATMs, Facebook, (Meta), Instagram, Twitter, Snapchat, TikTok and so on. Because humans are by nature gregarious, this disconnection and isolation has had a huge negative impact on mental health.

The fight response has resulted (for example) in increased domestic violence and government-funded ad campaigns telling us not to be angry.

With the advent of the COVID virus, anxiety and depression have increased dramatically, spurred on by mass and social media focused on propagating panic and fear. People are glued to their TV sets and radios waiting for, and listening to, the latest shock news. The propagation of bad news and negative views is great for TV and radio ratings.

# Why this guide?

There is not much we can do about the world out there, but we *can* do something about ourselves. It is not as difficult to deal with anxiety and depression as we have in many cases been led to believe, and taking a pill is usually not the answer! This guide is for people who have (or know people who have) been diagnosed with anxiety and/or depression and for those who just want to improve their general mental health. Anxiety is mostly caused by believing things that are not real. Depression is most often caused by an obsession with the past, which is dead, because it cannot be changed. As a result, we let something that is not real and is dead control our emotional state.

My intention is to offer help and practical, easy-to-follow suggestions to gain freedom from the prison of emotional pain by managing negative and self-limiting thoughts, which feed into the subconscious and are the underlying causes of mental health issues.

There are many types and degrees of anxiety and depression. For example, with depression, there is mild, non-clinical depression, major depression, melancholia, psychotic depression, ante and postnatal depression, bipolar mood disorders and so on. Parts of this book might be particularly relevant to you, so it's not a bad idea to read it with a highlighter!

*Remember:*

- We can easily learn the skills to manage our thoughts—it just takes practice.
- You don't know the future.
- You are more than your history.
- You are more than your symptoms.
- You have more resources than you realise.

# How to use this book

This book has two parts—*it is important to read part one as it makes part two more meaningful.*

## Part 1 - Understanding anxiety and depression

Understanding is an important part of healing. This part is about understanding in simple terms what we are dealing with and correcting some of the myths surrounding the emotional prison in which we can find ourselves.

## Part 2 - Taking action

This part is about taking action—acquiring the skills to manage our thoughts and retrain the way we think, and, in so doing, free ourselves from an emotional prison.

# Part 1
# Understanding anxiety and depression

# Thought-based symptoms of anxiety and depression

Understanding in simple terms what we are dealing with and challenging the myths surrounding our own emotional prison are both liberating and important, as once we understand the challenge, we can deal with it. It has a lot to do with our thoughts!

How do we know if we are what is labelled 'anxious' and/or 'depressed'? If we are, we might have some of these thought-based symptoms.[1]

---

1 Please don't read this list and automatically come to the conclusion that you have anxiety and/or depression. They are just indicators. If some of these symptoms are experienced to excess, (to the extent that they bother you,) then they become relevant.

# 1. Poor sleep

If a child has a bad night, they will often display negative emotions such as irritability, anger or tearfulness. Adults are no different. The following are examples of the sorts of thoughts that can deprive us of sleep.

- 'Must remember' or 'what if?' thoughts.
- Disturbing thoughts that cause us to have light sleep, often with distressing or excessively busy dreams, resulting in poor-quality sleep, so that we sometimes wake up after 8 hours of sleep but still feel tired.
- Thoughts (often inspired by poor planning) that cause us to get to bed late, such as, 'I must just finish this before I go to bed.'
- Thoughts that we might escape our thoughts by watching television in bed—a bad thing to do if we want quality sleep.
- Self-sabotaging thoughts, such as, 'I know I won't be able to sleep tonight.'
- Thoughts of regret, such as, 'If only I had done this, or that...'

# 2. Anxiety

This is a strong, frequently thought-based feeling of apprehension, worry or unease. For instance:

- Over-thinking, such as, 'I wish my mind would shut up.'
- Over-analysing, such as, 'I should have done this or that,' or, 'I wonder what she meant when she said that.'
- An overcrowded mind—too many thoughts sometimes causing confusion and panic and often resulting in poor memory and concentration.
- Indecisive thoughts—'I can't make up my mind.'
- Controlling thoughts—imagining that we can control what people are thinking about us, such as, 'People will think I'm stupid.'
- Negative 'what if?' thoughts that create scenarios about the future, which we can't possibly know. 'What if she did this? He would then do that and then this would happen.' A 'what if?' thought has no evidence—and yet we allow these unsubstantiated thoughts to control us. Often these thoughts come from an imagined future reinforced by past experience/trauma. (Positive 'what if?' thoughts such as, 'What if I go for a run? That might make me feel better' are overridden by negative 'what if?' thoughts when we are feeling low.)
- Thoughts of unfounded fears, such as, 'If I take my dog off the lead, he will run away and never come back or get run over by a car.' Of course, if you are in a city, that is a sensible thought, but if you are in an off-lead park, or in the bush, the thought can be unfounded. It's not about the dog—

it's about you! Pets pick up on our fears and can become anxious themselves.

- Thoughts of extreme fear or being totally overwhelmed by stress, resulting in panic attacks.

- Thoughts giving rise to a fear of not being able to control something that is beyond our control, such as, 'I hate flying, as I always think the plane will crash.'

- Thoughts of needing to know everything, such as constantly asking questions when we may not really care about the answer. (This is a sign of anxiety, but also irritating to those people who feel they have to respond to these seemingly endless and pointless questions. These questioners often fear or are uncomfortable with silence.)

Of course, anxiety can come from reality (the current environment). 'The bull is charging at me.' Who wouldn't be anxious!

# 3. Irritability and anger

These behaviours are frequently directed towards those who are close to us (partner, family, etc.) and usually constitute the 'fight' responses to anxiety.

Here are some examples of thought triggers causing anger.

- Even an innocent comment can sometimes trigger a thought (usually from past experience), leading to irritation or an instant angry outburst. These outbursts often seem beyond our control due to their suddenness and often we don't understand where they have come from.

- Oversensitivity often results in over-defensiveness, irritability and anger—for instance, when a person thinks that their self-esteem is being threatened or their ability challenged. Often this oversensitivity comes from jumping to unfounded conclusions.

- Thoughts that give rise to a feeling of anger at the loss or withdrawal of approval. An example might be a partner falling out of love for us or a boss demoting us.

- Angry thoughts arising from the frustration of not being able to control someone or something—not realising that the only person we can control is ourselves! (An example of this is road rage resulting from the need to control the traffic.)

# 4. Thoughts causing low motivation

This mainly refers to feeling disinclined to do things for ourselves. Here are some examples.

- Thoughts of procrastination that make us struggle to get things done, such as, 'It doesn't really have to be done now. I'll get around to it later, but first I want to do this.'
- Thoughts arising from poor self-esteem, such as, 'I'm not capable. It's all too hard.'
- Thoughts arising from poor sleep or tiredness, such as, 'I just can't do that today.'
- Thoughts of futility, such as, 'What's the point? If I do it, it won't make any difference,' and, 'Even if I try to do my work or study, I have fallen so far behind I'll never be able to catch up.'

# 5. Lowered mood

These are self-limiting, frequently victim-based thoughts that can make us feel sad, miserable, overwhelmed, and trapped. These thoughts are mostly inward looking. Here are some examples.

- Thoughts of inadequacy, such as, 'I'm a failure.'
- Thoughts of disconnection—'No-one understands what it's like. No-one cares.'
- Thoughts of guilt—'It's all my fault.'
- Thoughts involving negative judgements, such as, 'Only bad things happen to me.'
- Self-destructive thoughts, such as, 'I'm worthless,' or, 'This will never end.'
- Misguided thoughts of escape that can lead to addiction. For example, 'I need a drink', 'I need a hit', 'Alcohol relaxes me.' (Alcohol and drugs are significant causes of anxiety and depression.)
- Dangerous thoughts of escape—'My life is not worth living. People would be better off without me.'
- Disempowering thoughts of grief. For example, 'I will never recover from the loss of my mother.'
- Hurtful, self-analytical thoughts resulting from a failure to get approval, such as, 'They don't like me because I'm shy.'
- Self-limiting thoughts arising from the frustration of constantly trying to get approval from others, such as, 'Something is really wrong with me because whatever I do is not good enough for them.'

# 6. Low self-esteem

A symptom of low self-esteem is when we judge ourselves by what *we think* others think about us (often because we don't know who we are). Here are some examples.

- Thoughts feeding a need for approval. We all like approval, but these thoughts are more like a craving and often result in putting the needs of others way ahead of our own needs just to win approval or praise. (This is only a band-aid, and we continue to need more and more outside approval.)

- Thoughts of low self-value, such as, 'My opinion doesn't matter. I'm not good at anything.'

- Destructive, self-judgmental thoughts—'I'm ugly', 'I'm fat.' (These can lead to mental disorders like bulimia, anorexia nervosa and addiction to expensive and damaging cosmetic procedures.)

- Self-sabotaging thoughts of self-doubt, such as, 'I'll never be able to do that' or, 'Nothing good ever happens to me.'

*Remember that people with high self-esteem are not usually anxious.*

# 7. Social withdrawal from family and friends

Often the flight response to anxious thoughts prevents us from going out or keeping up with others.

Here are some examples.

- Thoughts of insecurity—'It's safer staying at home.'
- Thoughts of self-deprecation,—'I'm too fat to go out—people notice,' or, 'I'm not interesting—no-one will want to talk to me.'
- Inertia-induced thoughts resulting in the inability to do usually enjoyable activities—'I just can't be bothered to go out.'
- Thoughts of wanting to be alone with our depression—'I'm going to wrap myself up in my warm blanket of depression where I feel secure, because I'm used to it.'
- Thoughts involving a fear of change—'I know my depression—people don't want to talk to a depressed person. I'll just stay at home with my depression. It's too scary to think about what life would be like without it.'

# 8. Perfectionism

The perfectionist strives to be flawless and, as this is not achievable, he or she usually ends up with depression. Here are some examples.

- Thoughts that everything must be done perfectly.
- Thoughts of being a failure if it is not done perfectly.
- Thoughts of resignation, like, 'Even if I do it perfectly, it will still not be perfect', or, 'I won't be able to do it perfectly, so I won't try.'

# 9. Low libido

This is often a symptom of depression, which can be exacerbated by the side effects of antidepressants. Examples of these thoughts are:

- 'I'm just too tired.'
- 'I can't be bothered.'
- 'He/She won't be able to turn me on.'
- 'I don't/can't feel anything.'

# 10. Freeze response

This is when, instead of expressing our emotions arising from our thoughts, we push them down. We now know that suppressed emotions are stored in the body and can cause physical conditions, because the body can be seen as a mirror of the mind. Pain in the mind is frequently translated into pain in the body.[2] Suppression of emotions is often the reason behind conditions like fibromyalgia and irritable bowel syndrome.

Other typical physical symptoms of anxiety and depression are:

- constant tiredness
- changes in weight
- inflammation
- muscle pain and headache
- general tiredness and chronic fatigue syndrome
- frequent illness and low resistance to infection
- skin rashes and welts.

---

2 In Western Medicine, the mind and body are separated, whereas in other forms of medicine like Traditional Chinese Medicine (TCM), Japanese Kampo Medicine and Indian Ayurvedic Medicine, the mind is seen as inseparable from the body. This is slowly starting to change in Western Medicine, spurred on by a brilliant research paper by Dr George Engel from the University of Rochester Medical Centre titled *The Biopsychosocial Model,* written over 40 years ago, which puts forward the notion that illness is a combination of biological, psychological and sociological influences. In the intervening years this view has gained significant traction—albeit slowly!

# 11. Empowered by depression

People who are anxious and/or depressed often get attention from concerned family and friends who are keen to help, and this is used by some as a source of power. Frequently it starts out as attention seeking and moves into control and manipulation. Sometimes this power is motivated by thoughts of revenge, arising from perceptions of not being good enough, or favouritism of siblings, etc.

Thoughts include:

- 'I was never good enough to be noticed. Now I have your undivided attention.'
- 'My depression gives me power. I don't have to work or do anything, and people worry and fuss over me. I always get my way.'

# Non-thought-based feelings of anxiety and depression

People often say things like:

'I just lost it with my friend for no reason. She said something which, when I look back, was totally innocent, and yet I experienced a feeling of uncontrollable anger.'

'I was driving my nice car alone on an open country road on a beautiful day. I was on my way to visit a friend in Bendigo. Suddenly, for no apparent reason, I felt a wave of deep sadness come over me and the tears flowed.'

These emotions and others can be triggered by things like scenery, a piece of music, a film or a book, etc. Why is this?

Your incredibly powerful subconscious mind is very much like a computer, and it remembers and holds on to everything. Much of this is inaccessible to the conscious mind. We see something and it triggers a feeling resulting from a past incident or feeling lodged in the data base of the subconscious, but without the conscious memory of the incident. This is why seemingly inexplicable waves of emotion can appear to come out of nowhere. Sometimes the inexplicable emotion triggers a negative thought, which aggravates the emotion.

'Why am I sad? Am I going crazy?'

The power of the subconscious is dealt with in more detail later in this guide.

# What are anxiety and depression?

*So, what are anxiety and depression? It has a lot to do with our thoughts!*

There are many differing views about what anxiety and depression are, however, they are mostly a thought-based state of mind—a state of mind that has been induced by circumstances beyond our control. Anxiety and depression come from learnt programs emanating from the past and from which self-limiting thoughts have arisen. None of these programs comes from us. There are good programs and not-so-good programs, and anxiety and depression arise from the latter. *Because* these programs come from others, it's not our fault! Anything the conscious mind believes, thinks or accepts passes straight into the vast data storage of the subconscious. The path to healing is to change what we feed into the subconscious by creating new habits of thinking. If we don't do this, we can slide into deeper depression, which affects our decision-making strategies. When depressed, we make poor decisions and this in turn leads to deeper depression. Depression causes itself!

# The connection between anxiety and depression

*Is there a connection between anxiety and depression? Yes—a close one!*

If we feel anxious, we usually feel insecure. If we feel anxious and insecure, we usually have self-doubt (low self-esteem). If we are anxious, insecure and have self-doubt, we are likely to become socially withdrawn and struggle with motivation. This could hardly make us happy—and so it is easy to move into depression. (It is, however, possible to feel anxious without being depressed.)

# The power of thought

*Your thoughts are so powerful, and they go beyond your head!*

An instrument called a Magnetoencephalograph (MEG) measures brain activity/waves, which are thoughts, without touching the head. In the July 2017 edition of *Popular Mechanics*, Avery Thompson writes, 'Your innermost thoughts might not be so secret after all. At least if you're thinking them inside an MRI machine.' So, physics demonstrates that our thoughts radiate out beyond the physical head. *Telepathy is now scientific!* We don't yet know how far these thoughts travel, but there is plenty of empirical evidence to suggest that they travel vast distances—to the other side of the world and, who knows, maybe beyond? As an example, I had not contacted an old friend in South Africa for over four years. A few weeks ago, I felt an urge to call him. I checked the time difference with Melbourne and as I picked up my cell phone he called. Sure, coincidence is possible, but highly unlikely. We know that thoughts go beyond the physical body. It therefore follows that we *can manifest what we think.*

We are trillions of particles of energy and when we are attracted to people, these energy waves become intertwined. That's why we should be guided by these and not what other people say in relationships. We are thought generators sending out thought waves all the time. These thought waves resonate, with people sending out similar waves. However, if we are sending out waves of fear, a mugger is more likely to attack us than someone who is not sending out these waves.

If you are about to go into a room where you are due to be interviewed for a job, you have the power to influence the outcome.

You may choose to think negatively:

'There will be three people on one side of a table, and I will be on my own on the other side—they won't like me and they will ask me questions and I won't know the answer.'

These thoughts can be self-fulfilling because your thoughts go beyond your head and the interview could go badly.

You may choose to think positively:

'The interview panel will really like me and that's because I know what I am doing, and the interview will go well.'

There is a good chance that this will bring about a positive outcome. Because our thoughts go out beyond the physical body, they are subliminally picked up by others—in this case, the interview panel.

Positives attract positives and negatives attract negatives. This is also evident in the placebo effect. One third of all healing comes from the placebo effect—including surgery!

Patients with osteoarthritis of the knee who underwent placebo arthroscopic surgery were just as likely to report pain relief as those who received the real procedure, according to a Department of Veterans Affairs (VA) and Baylor College of Medicine study published in the *New England Journal of Medicine*, 12 July 2002. Conversely, the nocebo effect causes us to think ourselves into mental and physical illness. (The nocebo effect is the opposite of the placebo effect. It describes a situation where a negative outcome occurs because of a belief that the treatment will cause harm.) *So, positive thinking can heal you and negative thinking can kill you!*

Our thoughts can create our beliefs, and these can control our bodies and even defy science. Here are two examples: fire walkers walk over red-hot coals with no burns to the feet because they believe that they will be unharmed: some yogis can control and alter their blood pressure and temperature while sitting still.

If we can retrain the way we think, we change our beliefs and move from self-limiting to self-fulfilling thoughts—we can bring about the life changes that we want. It sounds simple, and it is! We must just practise!

# How did I come to be anxious and/or depressed?

Kenneth Kendler, M.D., Professor of Psychiatry and Genetics at the Medical College of Virginia, writes that 'the strongest predictor of major depression is still our life experience'. Contrary to what we are often told, there are no genes that make us depressed—it's all about the social environment or life experience we encounter, particularly in the early years of life. Recent research from US universities such as Boulder and McGill has demonstrated this and one of the studies from Boulder University involved a study of half a million people.[3]

There is so much that we are continuing to discover—there is even research indicating that our genes aren't permanent. Professor Bruce Lipton (with his work in the field of epigenetics) maintains that our genes, like our minds, can be affected or influenced by the environment surrounding them. For example, in a family where cancer is always being talked about, their genes can mutate towards cancer. Could this be the same with anxiety and depression? It certainly seems possible.

The notion that our thinking can influence our genetic make-up is a further reason why it is essential that we change the way we think, and this is the main purpose of this book.

---

3 See under References at the end of this book for a link to the work of Prof. Scott M Monroe from Notre Dame University in this field.

# Harmful subconscious programs

## The first seven years

In most cases, it all starts in the first seven years of life. The powerful computer-like subconscious is fully functional at birth and, during the pre-school years, it absorbs into its data base everything that occurs and unquestioningly takes on the programs from the surrounding social environment. The subconscious accepts everything that the conscious feeds it. In those early years, the conscious mind has no reference points or life experience, and therefore no judgement skills, so it blindly accepts what it observes and that information feeds into the subconscious programs and beliefs, where it is stored for life. That is why we are so vulnerable in those early developing years. There is evidence that the mind is even active during the last two months of gestation. It *cannot* experience touch, taste, smell, sight or sound, but it *can* sense mood and stress in the mother. This may explain why some babies are born stressed.

The subconscious mind is very easy to understand. It is incredibly powerful and very much like a supercomputer. And, like a computer, it simply accepts information fed into it by the conscious mind, without question, and holds onto it. If, for example, I type onto my computer that all cows have pink and green stripes, my computer simply accepts that information and stores it until such time as it is needed. Similarly, the young child with little or no life experience or judgement skills just observes, accepts and absorbs without judgement. This includes the good and the bad. All too often, for example, young children acquire addictive programs in the early years through watching and absorbing without filters or judgement. Some examples include the actions and behaviours of a parent or parents who use drugs, smoke, gamble and drink to excess. (These programs are worse when anger and bullying are combined with parental addiction to alcohol and drugs, especially methamphetamines.)

*The information capacity of the subconscious is so powerful that in those early years children can, for instance, easily learn three to five languages.*

From birth, a child takes in and accepts the behaviours and programs going on around her or him. If, for example, the child's mother or father is anxious or depressed, the child simply adopts that behaviour without question. Similarly, that child's parent or parents could have had an anxiety-causing start to *their* life/lives. That is why anxiety and depression can appear genetic, but they're not! Feeling loved and connected is vital for a child.

If attachment hasn't happened in the first two years, it can cause major problems later in life, such as with dependence, intelligence, anger, substance abuse, ADHD, depression, anxiety and more. I had an eight-year-old client who presented with high anxiety and some resultant disturbing OCD behaviour. She had a co-dependent, excessively needy relationship with her mother. Throughout her consultations, she didn't leave her mother's lap. She had an arm around her mother's neck and with the other arm, she clutched a fluffy toy to her chest. On questioning her mother, I found out that the child had been in care from the age of six months while her mother went to work. The child was highly stressed, clinging to her mother and in tears when being left at the day care centre.

This is a form of PTSD resulting from a lack of attachment in those crucial first two years. It seemed to me that the issue was not so much the disturbing OCD behaviour, but rather the little girl's lack of confidence resulting from an embedded subconscious feeling that she wasn't wanted. I suggested a program of confidence building involving the child taking tiny steps out of her comfort zone each day. These little steps were to be praised. The strategy worked, but it took time and patience. Six months later, the child was happier, more confident and the OCD behaviour had ceased.

There are many things in a child's early life that can cause anxiety, usually leading to depression. Some of these include:

- domestic violence—verbal and/or physical
- bullying
- disconnection—emotional, verbal or physical
- abandonment—emotional and/or physical
- emotional blackmail and manipulation
- fear of unpredictably quick-tempered parents
- financial stress
- micromanagement

Let us take the example of a young child (we will call her Suzie). Let's suppose that Suzie, for whatever reason, has acquired anxiety (which leads to depression) in her early years. She is now in the playground at primary school. Because she is in primary school, her life experience has been growing, and she is starting to be able to make judgements and is beginning to filter what she sees and experiences before it passes into her subconscious. She is learning a different way. Now she's learning by habituation—which is practice and revision. She witnesses an incident—for example, an older girl bullying a younger girl. Her computer-like subconscious mind then instantly scans her entire short life and connects to a past experience that relates to that bullying incident. Suzie then has a much stronger reaction to that incident than, say, Chloe, who has come from a calm, peaceful, nurturing and supportive background. So, despite her filtering ability, the bullying incident connects directly to the relevant stored information in her subconscious and triggers her reaction. That incident then becomes another trigger point in Suzie's life. As she gets older, there are more trigger points through which her subconscious scans. That is why in virtually all cases, when anxiety and depression start in the first seven years, they get worse as we get older. This is simply because there are more trigger points back through which the subconscious mind scans. Children in the first seven years are highly vulnerable to the programs that parents give them through their parenting.

We never get better if we see ourselves as victims, but in the early years we were victims simply because we didn't have a say in the programs to which we were subjected and we had no filters to protect us. *We can make or break our children in the pre-school years.*

Religious organisations know the power of mind programming in the early years.

'Give me the child for the first seven years and I will give you the man.'[4]

---

4 This is a quotation attributed to Ignatius Loyola, founder of the Jesuit movement in the Catholic Church. *The Catholic Doctrine of Original Sin* inspired by St. Augustine was formalised as part of Roman Catholic doctrine by the Councils of Trent in the 16th century.

The St Augustinian doctrine of Original Sin teaches that a child is born sinful—with 'the sins of the fathers'. It is a powerful tool for creating low self-esteem and insecurity and a resulting dependence on the church. A child is programmed to believe he or she is bad and must attend church and confess sins until the end of life. The congregation is endlessly told that it is sinful—it is in the Catholic Creed, repeated in every Holy Communion service. The biblical concept of the Devil and Eternal Damnation in Hell introduces fear very effectively in the innocent, accepting brain of the young child. It's not just the Catholics who use the power of these early years to amass congregations and wealth—most other religions do the same.

Mirror neurons (located mainly in the medial frontal and medial temporal cortex of the brain) cause us to imitate what we see. Mirror neurons make the child even more prone to absorbing and imitating these programs. This imitation can be nasty— for example, a young boy mirroring the behaviour of his father abusing his mother. A child who has experienced a bullying parent in the early years is far more likely to be a bully at school than one brought up in an equanimous family.

Anxiety and depression don't always start in the early years. We can have a nurturing, supportive and caring childhood and still become anxious and/or depressed later in life. This usually occurs as a result of a traumatic incident, which then becomes the Initial Sensitising Event (ISE). The trigger points can then start from that incident. These entrenched past experiences become the programs from which our thoughts arise.

What the conscious mind accepts can also be negated by powerful subconscious programs from the past. For example, people who endlessly read self-help books and/or attend high-priced events/programs presented by obscenely wealthy self-styled life-coach gurus get a real buzz or lift from the experience, but if the subconscious programs don't fit with the experience, within weeks, it is as though the event or experience didn't happen. For change to happen there has to be sustained practice. These 'wow factor' weekends are not enough.

# Same family, different experiences

How is it that two children in the same family, subject to the same programs, can sometimes grow up so differently?

One child could be highly anxious and the other sibling much calmer. Just as we have different physical pain thresholds, so we have different emotional pain thresholds. Some of us are more sensitive than others. This means that the same experiences can have different effects on siblings. For example, grief for a deceased parent can affect two siblings with very different intensities. (A first-born child is usually exposed to more anxiety than subsequent children simply because it is the first time for the parents.)

Two siblings growing up in the same family with the same environmental conditions are not affected in the same way. We perceive identical events differently and therefore they affect us differently. How often have you discussed a childhood event or experience with a sibling only to hear that sibling tell you, 'That's rubbish—it happened like this!' You and your sibling—with the aid of your powerful subconscious minds—each scan through all your individual past trigger points and view the same event differently because we experience everything differently and the way we view the past is often guided by our triggers.

Look at your fingerprints—no-one in the world has the same as you. We are all unique, and that is the problem when we are lumped into categories through labelling.

# The inner child

No matter how old we are, we always have an inner child. We grow up with different subconscious programs that form that inner child.

Think about your inner child.

- What sort of child is she or he? Happy? Sad? Insecure? Connected? Disconnected? Calm? Angry? Confident? (Remember that confident people are far less anxious.)
- What programs made your inner child like that?

# Relationships

The more we learn about the biology of depression, the more we discover the power of human relationships to either increase or decrease our susceptibility to depression. There is an exciting movement away from conventional psychiatry into Relational Psychiatry—recognising the role of relationships in mental health. One of the leaders is Dr Duncan Double, Consultant Psychiatrist at the Norfolk and Suffolk NHS Foundation Trust[5].

Unsatisfactory relationships are a major cause of depression. How often are other people at the heart of one's depression? Programs and thoughts resulting from an early history of disconnection, rejection, loss, betrayal, humiliation, abuse and abandonment all contribute to depression. Dr Michael Yapko says that 'regardless of culture, the people who are in positive, satisfying relationships, including in a relationship with themselves, do better in terms of mood and health'.

What is meant by being in a good relationship with ourselves? Take the example of a 22-year-old woman who has completed her studies and is working as a speech therapist. During her time of study, she has been in a relationship with a man and together they have saved and built a home. She is very creative, with a sense of adventure and wants to spend time travelling and working overseas before possibly settling down to a home life with children. Her partner is two years older and has his own plumbing business. He did much of the house building himself while his partner managed to study, work part-time and still offer manual building support whenever possible. Costs were shared equally, as

---

5 See under References at the end of this book for a link to his website.

she came from a wealthy family and her parents assisted. During the building of the home, both lived with their parents to save money. Recently, they moved into their home and his dreams were being fulfilled—owning his own home, having his own business, regularly seeing his mates and enjoying his sport, plus kids to come and an attractive partner to boot! He feels he is in a good relationship with himself.

She wants to rent the house out and travel but feels obliged to live the life he wants and become the housewife, mother and supporter of her partner in his business, social and sporting life. If she does this, she will start a poor relationship with herself and the consequences will be dire.

Being in like with someone generally lasts longer that being in love. Being in pity with someone is very easily confused with being in love.

Marital discord often leads to the thoughts that cause depression. Marital therapy can relieve this depression. How well our partner lives up to our expectations has a great impact on our degree of relationship satisfaction. What happens though if our expectations *aren't realistic*? How much of the anger, hurt and disappointment people experience in their relationships is a product of their own unrealistic expectations? In this case, the ability to love unconditionally and accept that no-one is perfect (including ourselves) is missing.

# Disconnection

Australia is one of the most prosperous countries in the world with one of the highest standards of living, and yet we are one of the world's poorest countries in terms of emotional health. I remember visiting African villages where the children had never heard of birthdays and had barely enough to eat. However, they were happy—playing together and making their own fun, making cars out of wire and guitars out of discarded oil cans, wire and wood, etc. They didn't know about anxiety, depression and suicide.

*Why is this not the case in Australia? Disconnection! They are connected and we are not.*

If a child's mother dies in the village, the child accepts it relatively quickly, because in the village, that child has many friends and family members. The children are forever visiting each other and having sleepovers in the huts of relatives and friends. They interact closely with siblings, aunts, uncles, grandparents, cousins and friends, which cushions their loss. They are connected! We are not. In the early years, parental and family attachment is vital for later emotional and mental health. These children are attached. In Australia, these essential attachment years are frequently missing, as both parents head off to work and hand their children over to strangers at day care.

Societies where the family unit is strong and where, for example the whole family gathers for Sunday lunch, tend to record a lower incidence of anxiety, depression and suicide.

*Disconnection causes anxiety and when this is fuelled by insecurity, it frequently leads to depression.*

In Australia we are even nervous about getting too close to our neighbours for fear that they might impose on us or become a problem. According to the 2016 census, more than two million Australians live in one-person households (which equates to 24% of Australian households). In addition, 16% of households are single-parent households, indicating that at least 40% of Australian households would have single parents or residents.

A child who grows up in a disconnected environment has a disconnection program. As an adult, that person usually has trouble forming long-term relationships because their program is about disconnection. Because these people are disconnected, they are also insecure and need constant approval. They often have affairs—not because they don't love their partner, but because the program won't allow the connection of a loving relationship. The flattery and attention of an affair can often overrule common sense and feed a desire for approval and connection and can leave behind broken hearts and broken families. It is an example of the conscious mind trying to appease the pain of a subconscious program and making bad choices.

# Fight, Flight and Freeze

Disconnection has made us an insecure society. Insecurity leads to anxiety and the related fight response has made us an angry country. It is simple. Disconnection causes insecurity, insecurity causes anxiety, and anxiety has three responses—fight, flight and freeze.

- *Fight*—Domestic and other anger-fuelled violence statistics in Australia continue to rise at a disturbing rate.
- *Flight*—The number of socially withdrawn people in Australia continues to grow, as does the number of people living alone.
- *Freeze*—The suppression of feelings and emotions is a cause of the growth of many physical conditions, such as fibromyalgia and irritable bowel syndrome.

# 'Fakebook'—social media and bullying

Social media can also be disconnecting. People in the 25–44 age group are the largest group of depression sufferers and, consequently, their children are the fastest-growing group of depressives (mainly because of the programs originating in *their* early years). Among young adults, depression is more common among the highest users of social media. Social media is actually disconnecting, because it replaces human contact and interaction with screen time and 'virtual friends'. Young people in Australia can frequently be seen in a group, out for coffee or a meal, and no-one is talking. They are all texting. Who are they texting? Often the very people at the table! Many young people would rather text than talk with a friend. They seldom answer phone calls, instead feeling safer by checking their message bank and texting back.

Why 'Fakebook'? Posts are frequently fake, creating photoshopped images, for example, of the perfect body and the flawless face, causing young people to believe what they see and to feel inadequate. 'Friends' post photos and accounts of highlights in their lives — holidays, romantic moments, etc. Followers believe that every day is like that for these people. It is fake—not real— and it damages self-esteem.

Researchers at Pittsburgh University surveyed 1,787 young adults aged 19–32 about their use of social media (Facebook, Twitter, Snapchat, Instagram, etc.) and administered a depression assessment. Respondents who reported the most social media use throughout their day were almost twice as likely to be depressed than those who reported the least use.[6]

6 *Association between Social Media Use and Depression among U.S. Young Adults,* Lin, Sidani, Shensa et al., 19 January 2016

Girls use social media more than boys and are more likely to report cyberbullying than boys, but it is interesting to note that it occurs more through texting and emailing than through Facebook or other social media websites. The majority of cyberbullying victims are also victims of school bullying. Teen bullying accounts for a large proportion of adult depression—frequently exacerbated, of course, by the trigger points dating back to the programs established in the early years.

A study of nearly 700 teenagers conducted by investigators who were led by Prof. Lucy Bowes at Oxford University showed that individuals who reported being bullied frequently at the age of 13 were about twice as likely to suffer from depression at the age of 18 — compared with their peers who did not experience bullying.[7]

Bullies have usually developed a subconscious bullying program as a result of being bullied themselves in their early years. An angry/violent father or mother can instil this program in the child —and bear in mind that those very parents are highly likely to have acquired a similar program from *their* parents.

While social media cause anxiety and depression, they also provide a powerful but potentially harmful vehicle that insecure young people can use to feed their growing need for approval— the 'look at me' syndrome in selfies, Snapchat, etc. Social media dating sites are frequently adorned with photoshopped images and this in turn creates the stress of the lie and the stress of trying to get through the resultant first date. Things like this can make young people vulnerable to bullying, ridicule and disapproval. Depression often follows when the approval is not forthcoming in the expected number of 'likes'.

---

7 Published online 2 June 2015 in the British Medical Journal. See under References at the end of this book for a link to an interesting interview with Prof. Bowes.

Sometimes depression is severe, leading to suicide. Over 65,000 Australians attempt suicide each year. In 2017, there were 3,000 suicides. Suicide is a leading cause of death of Australians between the ages of 15 and 44 and 75% of suicides are male. (This is because women tend more towards the 'cry for help' attempts than men.) More young Australians take their own lives than die in motor vehicle accidents (and this doesn't take into account the road deaths that may themselves have been unrecognised suicides).[8]

8 26 and 27 September 2017, Australian Bureau of Statistics.
http://www.abs.gov.au/Causes-of-Death

# Harmful conscious strategies

*Does the conscious mind do anything to help?*

Yes. The conscious mind can retrain the ingrained subconscious programs from the past, through repetition (habituation). The conscious mind wants to ease emotional stress. It is what makes us seek help.

Unfortunately, well-intentioned conscious mind strategies can be damaging. Here are six examples of harmful conscious mind strategies.

# Harmful strategy 1: being controlling

*'A jumper is something you put on when your mother feels cold!'*

Anxious people often appear controlling, but they are not inherently controlling at all—it's just a defence strategy of the conscious mind. The conscious mind is our friend—it wants good things for us — but it is not nearly as powerful as the subconscious, from which our programs emanate. The subconscious mind isn't good, and it isn't bad—it is just a computer and it holds onto everything that has been fed into it from early childhood, making no judgements. The conscious mind thinks:

> 'I can't take this anymore. My emotions arising from my subconscious programs are controlling me. What can I do? Oh, yes, I know! I can't control my feelings, but at least I can control and/or micromanage other people. That will give me some control.'

# Harmful strategy 2: causing an obsessive-compulsive disorder (OCD)

There are five common manifestations of OCD:

- A fear of contamination—resulting in obsessive washing
- Constant checking
- A strong desire for order and symmetry
- Rituals
- Hoarding

An obsessive-compulsive disorder is the same conscious mind strategy as the first harmful strategy outlined above. Anxiety makes us insecure. The conscious mind thinks:

'I can't take this anymore. My insecurity is controlling me. What can I do? Oh, yes, I know! I can't control my feelings of insecurity, but at least I can have order and pattern in my life.'

Order or routine gives the anxious person some certainty and this to some extent alleviates anxiety (which is often based on uncertainty). This search for certainty and confirmation can easily become obsessive.

The attempts of the conscious mind to find certainty can develop into repetitive checking and rechecking. People with an obsessive-compulsive disorder also tend to do things simply because they have always done them—it makes them feel secure—but, sadly, it is never enough. Your hands are never clean enough, the door is never going to be locked, the house will never be completely in order and, 'If I don't do this ritual before hitting the golf ball, it will always be a bad shot'. Often the compensatory act of repeatedly washing the hands comes from guilt (the Lady Macbeth effect—washing away the guilt). Hoarding is also a common feature of OCD—the need to collect or possess things comes from the need for security.

# Harmful strategy 3: causing weight issues

Overweight people often have low self-esteem and are anxious and/or depressed. As in the previous examples, the conscious mind might say:

> 'I can't take this anymore. My emotions are controlling me. What can I do? I need comfort. Oh, yes, I know! Eating (especially sweet or junk food) gives me comfort, so every time I have a disturbing thought and resulting emotion, I'll eat.'

This soon becomes an unhealthy habit.

# Harmful strategy 4: causing addictions

Again, it's the same as in the previous instances:

> 'My anxiety and low self-esteem are controlling me. What can I do? Oh yes, I know! I can't control my feelings of insecurity, but at least I can get drunk, or high, or gamble, or watch porn, or undergo cosmetic procedures, and that will give me a break from these feelings of inadequacy.'

# Harmful strategy 5: 'I'm better than you!'

We all want approval, but with low self-esteem, this need for approval is heightened and can lead to increased anxiety and unfortunate behaviour. People with low self-image often fight it by being judgmental and running others down. They look for and talk about the shortcomings of others so that they will look or feel better than the ones they are criticising. We can see this in the rapid growth in popularity of so-called 'reality TV', where —with almost voyeuristic delight—the audience witnesses the misfortunes of the participants, who in turn want approval by being on national TV, even if it is as a subject for derision (Dr. Phil, for example).

 Feeling like you are better than others becomes a conscious mind strategy to deal with a subconscious program of inadequacy. This can sometimes lead people to make poor financial decisions in an attempt to appear better than others. They might buy a brand-new expensive car instead of a year-old one. They might spend lavishly on designer labels. They might pay an exorbitant price or rent for a house or apartment just to be able to say, 'This is where I live.' They might indulge in expensive and painful cosmetic surgery just to have people comment on how young they look for their age—we take fat from our butts and put it in our cheeks! It is interesting to observe how many people (especially women) feel a subliminal compulsion to compete in clothing and looks with other women when they socialise. This is a significant contributor to anxiety levels.

It is sad that many doctors are injecting botulinum toxin (Botox —one of the most poisonous substances known) under the skin of both young and older people, who seek the temporary self-image boost of looking good—until their next three-monthly injection. Botulinum toxin is a neurotoxin causing muscular paralysis. Its composition and administration have to be carefully undertaken and that is why doctors or nurses (who have had special training by doctors) administer it. But why? You decide. For the long-term wellbeing of their patients? I wonder. Long-term efficacy and effects are often very different from initial expectations. Cosmetic procedures, including surgery, frequently become addictive, as constant improvement is sought in the seemingly never-ending quest for approval (and to the financial delight of many cosmetic surgeons)!

# Harmful strategy 6: getting approval at all costs

Similarly, in an effort to alleviate low self-esteem, the conscious mind can cause us to go out of our way to please others to the extent that we forget about our own needs—just to get others to like us. We end up living our lives for others.

In Anita Moorjani's inspirational book *Dying to Be Me* (2012), she describes how, when all hope of recovery from her lymphoma was gone and the medical profession had given up on her, she had a near-death, out-of-body experience in which she realised that her whole life had been spent trying to please others and not herself, and that this was actually killing her. When she came back into her body, she was transformed—one of those experiences that we can't account for, but that does happen. She left the hospital totally free of cancer and has been free of cancer ever since. This book is worth reading. There are thousands of cases throughout the world where people have been told that there is no chance of recovery and that they should go into palliative care, and they suddenly defy all medical science and (seemingly) inexplicably get better. Doctors call this 'spontaneous remission' because it can't be medically explained. What we do know is that spontaneous remission usually occurs after a positive shift in thought, circumstances, or attitude.

While the above strategies list some of the well-intentioned, but detrimental effects of the conscious mind's attempts to help, it is important to recognise that the conscious mind does great things too. It is a filter that comes between an experience and the computer-like subconscious, which just accepts and stores information. Remember that whatever the conscious mind accepts goes straight into the subconscious without question.

*So, with practise we can bring about change in the subconscious through creating new habits of conscious thinking and, in so doing, change the self-limiting messages we send to the subconscious.*

# A word on medication

## Is there a place for antidepressant and anti-anxiety medication?

*Yes. However, they should not be the sole treatment—and all too frequently they are!*

Antidepressant and anti-anxiety medication are essentially tranquilisers and may have some value in the short term in suppressing or blunting the intensity of mood and emotion. They could form a steadying base on which coping strategies can be built, but they are not a cure in themselves and are overused. They also have a place in the case of people who have an excessive fear of change. Their depression has been pervasive for as far back as they can remember—it's all they have ever known. The thought of being without medication is worse than the condition itself and they feel comfortable being tranquilised. The tranquilisers give them a sense of security. In those cases, the placebo effect is paramount—as is so eloquently demonstrated in Professor Irving Kirsch's brilliant book, *The Emperor's New Drugs: Exploding the Antidepressant Myth*, (published by Basic Books).

I am not a fan of antidepressants or anti-anxiety medication for many reasons, and it is likely that many in the medical profession will disagree with my opinion. My purpose is simply to open your mind to the very real possibility that what you have believed about anxiety and depression might not be true. In the interests of credibility, I have quoted eminent health practitioners and academics. It is not difficult to understand, and I urge you to read through what follows.

We are often told that anxiety and depression are genetic. No such gene has been found. In contrast there is much evidence that it is environmental. We are also told that a lowering of the serotonin levels in the brain is a major cause of depression and anxiety. This is called into serious doubt by many leading academics and health practitioners.

*Here is some of this evidence.*

The National Centre for Health Statistics in the US reported that the rate of antidepressant use in teenagers and adults (particularly Selective Serotonin Reuptake Inhibitors—commonly abbreviated as SSRIs) increased by 400% between 1998–1994 and 2005–2008. Australia has one of the highest rates of antidepressant use in the world. Fifteen per cent (1 in 8) of Australians take them daily and use in children has increased proportionally. The use of antidepressants in Australia has more than doubled since the year 2000, despite evidence showing that the effectiveness of SSRIs is highly doubtful.

Dr Michael Yapko, a leading world expert on depression, wrote:

'As we are learning the hard way because of deception, misdirection and the power abuses of the pharmaceutical industry, antidepressants are not nearly as effective as we have been led to believe.'

His view gained Australian academic support in an article published in the *Medical Journal of Australia*, May 2016 by C. Davey and A. Chanen, titled 'The unfulfilled promise of antidepressant medications'.[9]

---

9 See under References at the end of this book.

All the findings from this article were highly concerning, but for the purposes of this book, the most relevant findings on the ineffectiveness of antidepressants were:

- the unfortunate messages coming from many health professionals—'You don't have to change your life, you don't have to learn new skills, *you just have to take your medication on time.*'

- pseudoscientific, false advertising—for example, serotonin deficiency is a heavily promoted theory with little empirical support and considerable contradictory evidence.

- drugs are overprescribed.

- side effects such as weight gain can be more than just an irritant. In fact, some side effects can reduce or prevent participation in treatment, complicate symptoms and serve to reinforce depression and in some cases even lead to suicide.

- the therapeutic efficacy of antidepressants is in grave doubt —*this issue alone makes all the other concerns secondary.*

The famous STAR*D Study (Sequenced Treatment Alternatives to Relieve Depression) was set up by the US National Institute of Mental Health in 2006, involving 4,041 outpatients between 18 and 75 years of age and run over seven years. It found that 67% of patients on antidepressants did feel an improvement, but that within a year, half of them were fully depressed again. Only one in three showed a lasting improvement—but bear in mind *that number included those people who would have recovered naturally without the pills.*

## Chemical imbalance — fact or myth? You decide!

Because people are being told by many in the medical profession that their problems stem from a chemical imbalance in the brain, it may be a good idea to question this. Being told that your problems are chemical is disempowering as you are told that fighting this with SSRIs like Lexapro, Zoloft, Prozac, etc., is the only way. Many eminent scholars and respected academics call this theory into doubt. Here are the views of some of them. Take the time to read what they have to say and make up your own mind.

### Professor David Healy

Writing in the British Medical Journal in 2015, David Healey, Professor of Psychiatry at the Hergest psychiatric unit at Bangor University in North Wales points to a misconception that lowered serotonin levels in depression are an established fact, which he describes as, 'the marketing of a myth'. He maintains that low serotonin is a mythical cause of depression, and he is highly skeptical of the efficacy of SSRIs, which include drugs such as:

- Fluoxetine (Prozac or (Sarafem)
- Fluvoxamine (Luvox)
- Citalopram (Cipramil)
- Sertraline (Lustral)
- Paroxetine (Seroxat)
- Escitalopram (Cipralex)
- Vortioxetine (Brintellix)
- Lexapro
- Zoloft.

I recommend that you watch interviews with Professor David Healy on YouTube. He believes that we are taking far more drugs for everything than we should be. His argument is strong and worth listening to.[10]

(Prof. Healy is also author of many revealing books including *Let Them Eat Prozac: The unhealthy relationship between the pharmaceutical industry and depression.*)

## Dr Philip J. Cowen

*Serotonin and depression: pathopsychological mechanism or marketing myth?* is a fascinating article by Philip J. Cowen, neuroscientist in the Department of Psychiatry at Oxford University, published in 2008 in the journal, *Trends in Pharmacological Sciences* (Elsevier).

His article concludes with this statement:

> Simple biochemical theories that link low levels of serotonin with depressed mood are no longer tenable.

## Ronald W. Pies MD

Dr Pies is Professor in the psychiatry departments of SUNY Upstate Medical University, Syracuse, NY and Tufts University School of Medicine, Boston and past Editor in Chief Emeritus of *Psychiatric Times*. In his article, published on April 30, 2019, he concludes:

> In the 1980s, the 1990s, and beyond, pharmaceutical companies heavily promoted something resembling a chemical

---

10 See under References at the end of this book for more on over-prescription. (Prof. David Healy)

imbalance theory of mood disorders directly to consumers —or, at least, used the 'chemical imbalance' trope to explain how antidepressants supposedly work. In recent years, as psychologist Dr John Grohol (founder of Psych Central) has *pointed out*, some non-professional websites have provided misleading graphics that reinforce the 'chemical imbalance' trope. It is not surprising that the 'Theory That Never Was' has taken hold in the minds of so many.

## What about serotonin and anxiety?

More than 100 million people worldwide take SSRIs such as Prozac and Zoloft, to treat depression, anxiety and related conditions, but these drugs have a common and mysterious side effect: they can worsen anxiety in the first few weeks of use, which leads many patients to stop treatment. Scientists at the University of North Carolina (UNC) School of Medicine have mapped out a serotonin-driven anxiety circuit that may explain this side effect.[11]

## What about children?

If you have children, you might be aware that there is an alarming trend in recent times for medical and mental health professionals to prematurely diagnose and prescribe psychotropic drugs for children. Thankfully, many health experts have recognised this rush to diagnose and prescribe. Here are some examples which you might find illuminating.

---

11 See under References at the end of this book for an article entitled *How do antidepressants trigger fear and anxiety?* (University of North Carolina Medical School)

59

## Dr J.N. Jureidini

Below are two extracts from an editorial published in the *Australian Prescriber* (October 2005) entitled *Suicide and Antidepressants in Children* written by Dr J.N. Jureidini, Psychiatrist at the Women's and Children's Hospital in Adelaide. He has also trained in philosophy (PhD, Flinders University), critical appraisal (University of British Columbia), and psychotherapy (Tavistock Clinic). Summarising his editorial and referring to antidepressants, he writes:

So, we have poor evidence of efficacy, small but significant increases in suicide risk, and significant, probably underestimated, adverse events. The evidence therefore shows us that antidepressants are not demonstrably 'better than nothing' and may be worse. This conclusion will be at odds with many general practitioners' clinical experience in using these drugs. The discrepancy arises because prescribers who have seen apparently positive responses to antidepressants have not realised that much of the observed benefit would have occurred in response to a placebo.

He concludes:

Recent recommendations from the UK National Institute for Clinical Excellence confirm that antidepressants are not appropriate for the treatment of mild depression in any age group. Their proposed strategy of 'watchful waiting' is appropriate for children with mild to moderate depression. Where acute risk is low, a general practitioner might offer a brief explanation about depression, sleep hygiene, the usefulness of finding a confidante, the benefits of exercise and of gradually resuming any activities set aside because the individual is 'too depressed'. The general practitioner should then arrange to see the patient again in about two weeks but offer to talk to them earlier if they are worried.

In more severe cases, referral to or consultation with a child and adolescent mental health service or a child psychiatrist is recommended. The limited availability of such services is an indication for advocacy; it does not mandate prescribing against available evidence. Such prescribing, based on faith or hope that antidepressants may actually be better than the evidence indicates, risks contravening the injunction to 'first do no harm'.

## Professor Joseph M. Rey

Joseph M. Rey, Professor of Child and Adolescent Psychiatry, Northern Clinical School, University of Sydney, in the same edition of the *Australian Prescriber* (above), writes:

When treatment with SSRIs (Selective Serotonin Reuptake Inhibitors which include drugs such as Lexapro, Zoloft, Prozac, etc.) is begun, the patients (and their families when appropriate — for example in younger adolescents) must be informed of the risk of increased suicidal thoughts and attempts, and adverse effects, so that they can detect 'activation', a manic switch, or an increase in suicidality, as well as discussing practical ways of dealing with them and enhancing patients' safety. This may require a reduction of the dose, because the adverse effects can be dose related. It is imperative to review patients often and monitor them closely for adverse effects, particularly during the first few weeks of treatment.

## A different view on ADHD

The misdiagnosis of ADHD has become far too common and therefore medication has been inappropriately overprescribed. The work of a truly brilliant psychologist, the late Jerome Kagan exposed this.

## Emeritus Professor Jerome Kagan

Jerome Kagan was an eminent American psychologist, Daniel and Amy Starch Research Professor of Psychology, Emeritus at Harvard University, and co-faculty at the New England Complex Systems Institute. He was one of the key pioneers of developmental psychology. In fact, his fellow academics ranked Kagan the 22nd most eminent psychologist of the 20th century. (This ranking put him ahead of *Carl Jung*, who was ranked 23rd!)

The following comments and quotes come from an article by Professor Kagan and published by the *Mental Health Empowerment Project* in the US on January 21, 2016.

> ...(ADHD) is an invention. Every child who's not doing well in school is sent to see a paediatrician, and the paediatrician says: 'It's ADHD; here's Ritalin.' In fact, 90 percent of these 5.4 million (ADHD-diagnosed) kids don't have an abnormal dopamine metabolism. The problem is, if a drug is available to doctors, they'll make the corresponding diagnosis.

He went on to say:

> If you do interviews with children and adolescents aged 12 to 19, then 40 percent can be categorized as anxious or depressed.

But if you take a close look and ask how many of them are seriously impaired by this, the number shrinks to 8 percent.

Professor Kagan also made the point that most children diagnosed with ADHD fall under one umbrella.

Who's being diagnosed with ADHD? Children who aren't doing well in school. It never happens to children who are doing well in school. So, what about tutoring instead of teaching?

Referring to the US, he said that misdiagnosis—and hence over-diagnosis—occurs across an entire spectrum of mental health conditions. In simple terms, not everyone who displays a symptom or behaviour has a mental health problem, especially children, who are prone to unpredictability.

Misdiagnosis leads to over-diagnosis, which is—in Kagan's view—a problem plaguing the mental health profession. Looking at the number of children diagnosed with ADHD, it is difficult to disagree. According to the United States Centre for Disease Control and Prevention (CDC), 'Approximately 11% of children 4–17 years of age (6.4 million) have been diagnosed with ADHD as of 2011.'

He concluded that mental health professionals must shift their approach to diagnosing ADHD, depression, anxiety, and other disorders. The answer? Psychiatrists and other mental health professionals need to begin making diagnoses similar to how most other doctors do: by looking at the causes, not just the symptoms. This is especially the case with children, who often don't have a great ability (or desire) to fully explain themselves.

It is important to remember that antidepressants don't help people to develop the key skills to enable them to live effectively.[12] No amount of medication can teach us:

- how to manage thoughts
- how to build and maintain a support network
- how to create healthier relationships
- how to heal the wounds of the past
- how to create more effective decision-making strategies
- how to build a realistic and motivating future
- how to solve problems
- how to selfheal and cope more effectively
- how to think more clearly and use judgement skills.

---

12 I don't recommend that clients come off antidepressants or anti-anxiety medication without consulting the prescriber or until something has been put in their place (like new habits of thinking), enabling the automatic management of unhelpful thoughts.

# Changing ingrained subconscious programs

### It's not anxiety or depression — it's just Mabel and Kevin!

It's not a good idea to wear labels. I sometimes suggest to my clients that we rename anxiety and depression and call them 'Kevin' and 'Mabel'. It works well because it takes the sting out of those sombre labels.

Labels exacerbate depression—often a diagnosis of anxiety and/ or depression is enough to make us more depressed! We start to doubt ourselves, sometimes even Googling the symptoms and making them fit us! Anxiety and depression are simply intimidating labels for collections of negative and self-limiting thoughts. In most cases you can't feel sad, angry, worried, or indeed any emotion without first having a thought. (Sometimes we are not aware that we have had a thought because it happens so fast, coming up through a connecting trigger from a past experience.) So, anxiety and depression should be viewed as a label for our negative thoughts rather than a disorder or mental illness. Our thoughts are self-fulfilling, so, if most of our thoughts are positive, we are unlikely to be depressed or anxious.

### How do we know we can change ingrained subconscious programs?

After our early years we learn by conscious habituation—practice and revision—such as 'one times two is two, two times two is four', etc. So, if we have innocently acquired a limiting subconscious

65

program when young, the only way we can change that program later in life is by creating a new habit or way of thinking in the conscious mind and, through habituation (practice), alter these programs. Remember that the subconscious just accepts what the conscious feeds through. So, if we consciously create new habits of thinking, then with habituation (practice), these new habits filter through to the subconscious and change those self-limiting programs from the past.

The conscious mind is the creative mind: it can imagine things and create strategies. It wants good things for us, So, the way to bring about change is to practise, practise and practise!

For most of the day, we are being run by the subconscious mind. It is our autopilot! Have you walked down a street, talking on your phone with your thoughts miles away? Your subconscious walking program is taking care of everything so that you are not bumping into people, crashing into light poles, etc. Have you ever driven through a town and not remembered doing that? That's because the driving program in your subconscious was driving while your conscious thoughts were miles away.

If you were to hire a car in France, for instance, and had to drive on the other side of the road, your subconscious driving program would be disastrous—you would be in an accident in no time. Therefore, to drive in France you have to drive with your conscious mind—and it's really difficult because your conscious mind has to drop its wandering thoughts and concentrate on every detail. However, after a few weeks of regular practice, your conscious mind retrains your subconscious mind through practice (habituation), till eventually you are driving with a new program and with the same ease with which you drove at home.

That's very good news because we know we can change old habits of thinking! We *can* change our old self-limiting programs and generate new thought patterns, which in turn, brings us to emotional freedom. *Practice is the key!*

How long does it take to change our habits of thinking? With daily practice in most cases, four to six weeks. That's all! But it must be daily practice!

# Part 2
# Taking action

# How to take action

It is no coincidence that the therapies with the greatest success emphasise action in treatment. People dealing with depression may *feel* better in merely supportive therapy, but they will *do* better in treatment with direction. What follows is all about taking action to help ourselves and the other special people in our lives, including our children. I'm not suggesting that you should implement all of these strategies and suggestions for action—select those that best suit your situation and state of mind and start to practise them.

# Helping others

## Helping others — children

*How can we understand and help our children under threat of depression or anxiety?*

If a child is in those vulnerable early years (under the age of seven), the most important thing we can do is to make sure that we are giving the right signals — that we are being the best possible role model for our children in order to give them the greatest chance in life. The word 'educate' comes from *educo*, which is Latin for 'lead out or draw out'. We *lead* our children so that they are ready to go *out* into the wide world with confidence. Our purpose as parents is to support our children, especially in the early years, and prepare them for independence, so that they can live contented lives long after we are no longer around. Children are hardwired for struggle when they get here. Our job is not to see our children as perfect, but rather to prepare them for life and for their own imperfections.

*We create the programs in the early years that largely determine the mental health of our pre-school children in later life.*

Remember that children:

- have a wonderful imagination and think big
- like to know where they stand
- are by nature impulsive
- want what they want
- have a limited range of experience.

Children should not be micromanaged: they need to learn how to solve problems, how to evaluate alternatives, and how to understand consequences of actions and behaviours.

## Become the connected family

Disconnection in early life is a major cause of anxiety and depression in later life — take action. Here are some suggestions.[13]

- If you sense there is a problem, take prompt action. Don't wait.
- Create an environment for communication to occur.
- Listen non-judgmentally.
- Ask open-ended questions — 'Tell me about your school excursion', not 'How was your school excursion?' (The latter will invariably elicit a one-word answer: 'good'.)
- Where appropriate, ask for other interpretations of whatever has happened: 'Can we look at it another way?'
- Encourage physical activity.
- Encourage frequent social contact (not media).
- Seek out opportunities for fun.
- Encourage relaxation.
- Encourage self-care and taking personal responsibility.
- Contact a sleep talk consultant if you are worried about your child and use the techniques of sleep talk.[14]

---

13 Adapted from *Hand-Me-Down Blues* by Dr Michael Yapko

14 A very good Sleep Talk consultant is Kim High www.familyhypnotherapy.com.au

## Encourage regular bonding habits and build confidence

These strategies will enhance the connecting suggestions above.[15]

- Have meals together, share storytelling, do projects and take recreation together.
- Use familiar places for social interaction—kitchen, veranda, holiday place, etc.
- Encourage interests like sport, art, music and hobbies.
- Celebrate together—birthdays, achievements, a new job, etc.
- Encourage connection—visiting family and friends, family reunions, etc.
- Do storytelling about family history, members, ancestors, events; look at photographs together.

## Helping others—young adults

In recent times more and more depressed young adults are living in a shrinking world—staying at home often deep into their twenties, locked in their untidy cyber rooms. They don't work and seem oblivious to the effect they are having on themselves, their parents and family. It can sometimes help to give the person a reality check—explain that, as young adults, they have a choice, and no-one can make it for them. There are two pathways—continue as they are or change and start to make a life for themselves.

---

15 Adapted from *The Shelter of Each Other* by Mary Pipher, Ph.D.

Below is a typical eight-step pattern of emotional and mental decline in a depressed young adult.

1. Ask the person which step in *Pathway 1* they are on right now.
2. Look at the corresponding number in *Pathway 2*.
3. Leave it to them to consider.

These steps come from experience in my practice. They are of course not definitive, but rather indicative, so there will be variations.

Sometimes these steps are exacerbated by marijuana, alcohol, and other drug use. If that's the case, I have added the marijuana-assisted decline in italics at the bottom of each step.

**Pathway 1—The eight-step pathway down.**

1. Leaving school. Still with friends. Active socially and physically. Thinking about jobs/study.
2. Having the odd 'choof' (weed), and maybe the occasional 'bump' of coke.
3. Living at home with parents. Starting to withdraw socially, playing less sport. Making no attempt at further education or finding employment. Starting to feel disconnected from friends who are moving ahead with their plans. Spending more time in cyberspace (social media and games, etc,). Having unhealthy sleep patterns—staying up all night and sleeping by day.

   *Bored and 'choofing' more weed.*

4. Motivation starts to decline with less physical exercise

and more time alone. Health declines, often with weight gain. Friends lose interest. Everything (like getting a job, a driver's licence, joining a gym or sports club) seems too hard and it's always someone else's fault. Room is a mess. Parents trying fruitlessly to help and feeling trapped, sad, frustrated and helpless.

*Compensating with more weed.*

5. Feelings of worthlessness start to come. Anxiety rises with negative self-limiting thoughts—often exacerbated by online bullying. Only feeling secure in the confines of the bedroom. With anxiety comes a belief in negative things that have no evidence—for example: 'I worry about what people are thinking,' 'If I apply for a job, I won't get it,' 'People will think less of me,' 'I'll never get a girlfriend because I have nothing to offer, and I'm not attractive,' 'My friends don't like me,' and so on.

*More weed compensation.*

6. The fight response to the anxiety sets in. Holes punched in walls; furniture thrown around. Parents terrorised. Medication prescribed by mental health hospital — not taken. Often, instead of the fight response, the flight response gets worse with near total social withdrawal.

*Excessive weed use can lead to paranoia. Stealing from parents/ family to feed the habit.*

7. Deep depression. A feeling of being trapped in a shrinking world. A feeling of being the victim. A feeling of self-loathing and anger. A feeling of helplessness and guilt for being a burden. Self-harm by cutting because the physical pain alleviates the psychological pain. Hospitalisation.

(More females cut than males. Often, it's a cry for help.)
Parents getting older and family struggling to cope.

*Drug-induced psychosis. (Marijuana is the main cause of this.) Police involved. Involuntary hospitalisation in a mental health institution. Later returned home.*

8. A feeling that life is pointless. Parents can no longer cope, or they die. Family disconnects. Suicidal ideation.

   *Further drug-induced psychoses. Paranoia increasing. Moods all over the place. Regarded as a danger to him/herself or to others.*

9. Hospitalisation, CTOs, depot medication. In and out of mental health facilities.

   *Diagnosis of schizophrenia or a schizoaffective disorder, for which there is no known cure. Strong antipsychotic medication like Chlorpromazine and Risperidone prescribed. Permanently institutionalised in a care facility.*

Below is an example of another pathway. The choice is theirs.

## Pathway 2—Eight steps up.

1. Leaving school. With friends. Active socially and physically. Thinking about jobs/study.

2. Keeping up with friends and sporting activities/exercise. Applying for jobs or further study.

3. Meeting new friends and forming good relationships. Taking career and study opportunities. Leaving home. Keeping up with parents and family. Keeping fit and healthy. Saving for travel, car, house.

4. Getting promotion at work. Feeling valued and confident.

Finding a life partner. Spending six weeks touring Europe with partner and friends.

5. Getting a first home-buyer's grant and building or choosing a house. Winning the local basketball competition with teammates.

6. Moving into the new house with life partner. Very happy relationship. Accepting a new and attractive managerial job offer with exciting prospects.

7. Birth of first child and another planned.

8. Long service leave and joining friends on a caravan trip round Australia.

It's a matter of choice—is it time to cross to *Pathway 2*? Start by taking small steps. Ask this simple question each day:

'What can I do today that's different from yesterday?'

The answer could, for example, be:

- 'I can take the dog for a walk.'
- 'I can tidy my room.'
- 'I can phone a friend and catch up for a coffee.'
- 'I can join the local basketball team, where some of my old schoolmates play.'
- 'I can go on the net and see what jobs are available,' and so on.

The choice is theirs. It's not a dress rehearsal—it's real and the longer the decision is delayed, the harder it is to change.

## Helping others—adult family members and partners

It is not easy living with someone who is depressed and/or anxious. Here are some strategies and thoughts for help and support:

- Don't blame the person for being depressed.
- See the depression as a series of thought patterns to be shifted.
- Avoid clichés like, 'Cheer up,' 'Get a grip on yourself,' 'Pull yourself together,' and, 'Stop feeling sorry for yourself.'
- Don't try and 'save' the person from doing things they can do for themselves.
- Don't attribute the anxiety or depression to motivation problems—the anxiety and depression cause the low motivation.
- Getting out of anxiety and depression involves taking a series of small steps that require your encouragement.
- Focus on present challenges—there's no need to bring up past failures.
- The anxiety and/or depression is their problem, but not their fault in most cases. It comes mostly from programs in the subconscious emanating from the past—and these programs come from others.
- Don't feel guilty, but do what you can to help.
- Keep your own life going—if you don't, you can't help.

# Effective ways to address the social aspects of anxiety and depression

Social withdrawal is a part of anxiety and depression. Things to encourage are:

- Connections with others, especially with positive-thinking people.
- A sense of social responsibility to others, especially to partners and children.
- A habit of being outward-looking and having empathy.
- The habit of observing and accepting without judgement.
- Social action rather than analysis and self-analysis.
- Social contributions and acts of kindness.
- Thinking and behaving proactively.

# Helping ourselves

When we understand that depression is not a mental illness, that it is not genetic and probably not our serotonin levels, but rather a subconsciously induced state of mind, and that we can retrain our subconscious programs, we are ready for action and already beginning to heal.

Below are 36 strategies to improve the way we think and bring us to emotional freedom. I am not suggesting that all are relevant to your particular needs—you will find the ones that are most related to your situation. You may only need a few!

# 36 ways to change the way we think and improve our mental health

1.  What is my problem?

2.  Take exercise.

3.  Look outward, not inward.

4.  Challenge self-limiting thoughts and move on!

5.  Don't try to do the impossible—you are not perfect.

6.  Just accept and smile!

7.  Avoid jumping to conclusions.

8.  Goal setting—take small steps towards your goal.

9.  Avoid disconnecting habits.

10. Step outside your comfort zone.

11. Become socially connected.

12. Set aside a time to worry.

13. Get quality sleep.

14. Become the observer and healer—not the victim.

15. Mindfulness, meditation and hypnosis.

16. Hypnotise yourself and build expectancy.

17. A word about addiction.

18. Let go of your guilt.

19. Avoid uncertainty.

20. Imagine your perfect day.

21. Don't fear change.

22. Avoid mainstream and social media.

23. What about grief?

24. Stop being the judge and micromanager and let go of the need to control.

25. What about my work?

26. Avoid words of control.

27. Take control over how much you eat and lift your self-esteem.

28. Manage your anger and anxiety by replay.

29. Listen to your voice and to your speech habits.

30. Anti-freeze.

31. Dissociate yourself.

32. Talk to your inner child.

33. Cherish your experiences.

34. Be kind.

35. Breathe through your nose.

36. Count your blessings!

# 1. What is my problem?

There is a wonderful Neurolinguistic Programming (NLP) technique that requires us to answer this question, but we are *only allowed one word!* It requires some thought, but if we can reduce our issues and problems down to one word, it is highly therapeutic. It reduces our sea of self-limiting thoughts down to just *one word.* It gives us focus. One word is far better than a mass of thoughts. (Hypnosis is another useful tool to make that focus easier.) Once you have that one word, you will find it so much easier to heal and to see which of the strategies that follow might assist you.

# 2. Take exercise.

Physical exercise has the same effect as antidepressants, but without the side effects. Regular aerobic exercise (walking, swimming, riding, etc.) is an important step towards healing. When our thoughts are causing us to feel flat and demotivated, it can be very hard to motivate ourselves to exercise, but we *must* make that effort. When we exercise, we get our muscles and organs working efficiently: we get a healthy dose of mood-lifting dopamine into the brain and we take in more energy-giving oxygen.

There was a fascinating experiment led by Dr Michael Babyak, Professor of Psychiatry and Behavioural Sciences at Duke University in the US in 2000. It was conducted over three weeks with 156 people diagnosed with depression. They divided them into three groups. Group 1 exercised for half an hour, three times a week. Group 2 took an SSRI (Zoloft). Group 3 took Zoloft in the same dosage as Group 2 and they also did the same amount of exercise as Group 1. They found that Group 1 (exercise only) were 15% better than Group 3 (exercise and Zoloft) and 30% better than Group 2 (Zoloft only).

Charles H. Hillman, erstwhile Professor of Community Health at the University of Illinois and currently at the Northeastern University College of Science, found in a series of trials done in 2008 that aerobic exercise also improves cognition. These findings were published in 2008 in a journal called *Nature Reviews Neuroscience*. This article examines the positive effects of aerobic physical activity on cognition and brain function, at the molecular, cellular, systems and behavioural levels.

Here is an extract:

An emerging body of multidisciplinary literature has documented the beneficial influence of physical activity engendered through aerobic exercise on selective aspects of brain function. Human and non-human animal studies have shown that aerobic exercise can improve a number of aspects of cognition and performance. Lack of physical activity, particularly among children in the developed world, is one of the major causes of obesity. Exercise might not only help to improve their physical health but might also improve their academic performance. A growing number of studies support the idea that physical exercise is a lifestyle factor that might lead to increased physical and mental health throughout life.

In an Australian study of middle-aged depressed women, those who averaged 150 minutes of moderate exercise (golf, tennis, swimming, dancing, etc.) or 200 minutes of walking every week had more energy, socialised more, felt better emotionally, and weren't as limited by their depression. The study was over a period of three years.[16]

So, indeed, exercise is the best antidepressant!

16 K. Heesch, Y. van Gellecum, N. Burton et al. (online 13 January 2015), Australian Journal of Preventive Medicine

# 3. Look outward, not inward.

Avoid analysis paralysis—look outward, not inward. Anxious and depressed people tend to look inward, instead of at what's out there. If we are in a good mental state, looking inward can be a positive experience, but when we are depressed or anxious, we look inward negatively with destructive self-judgements and see ourselves as victims. (The Western World has become inward looking with guilt, blame and anger.) These inward thoughts are generally self-analytical, self-critical, self-sabotaging and self-limiting.

In addition, when we look inward, it's about us—and to friends and family it can appear like self-obsession as we play the victim. Remember that as long as we see ourselves as victims, we will not get better. Depressed victim-minded people can have many concerned friends trying to help, and they want that attention. But it's also important to realise how close the emotions of pity and love are. Do we want pity? I think not!

It's easy to test if you're self-obsessed. Look at the language you use.

- Notice how often you use the word 'I'. In other words, how often do you talk about yourself? There is nothing wrong with talking about yourself if it is of interest to others, but it is a question of balance.

- Are you forever turning the conversation towards yourself? For example, someone might be telling you or a group of friends about an event. They might say something that you can relate to, and instead of waiting till they finish, you interrupt and start talking about the same thing or something similar that happened to you.

- Are you uncomfortable with silence?
- Do you feel you have to fill every space?
- Do you say 'I...um...' before you think about what you're going to say? (I call this the 'I-yum syndrome'!) In other words, your first thought about filling that silence is filling it with something about you.

Self-obsession can often cause disconnection and we can lose friends. This disconnecting behaviour can stem from a combination of looking inward, needing attention/approval and becoming obsessed with a desire to be relevant.

Instead of looking inward, it's a good idea to look at the world out there *and listen to others*. We then cease to wilt and start to grow. How can we deal with this inward-looking habit? Create a new habit. When you start to feel an uncomfortable emotion, say, 'STOP! Am I looking inward or outward?' If the answer is inward, let the thought go because it is damaging you. Reduce the number of times you use the words 'I' and 'me'. Don't forget, if we are not in a good emotional state, when we look inward, we usually see ourselves as victims.

# 4. Challenge self-limiting thoughts and move on!

In the vast majority of cases, depression is caused by self-limiting thoughts arising from past programs, which in turn have arisen from our experience of negative past events, such as traumas, bereavements, regrets and guilt. Remember—it was what it was, and nothing can change that. The past is therefore dead energy. And yet, we let it control us with self-limiting thoughts. Instead of letting something which is dead control us, we can change how we react. We can't erase the memory, but we can remove the power that the memory exerts over us. Past trauma doesn't describe *who* we are. For example, don't say, 'I am an abuse survivor'. That's a dangerous self-limiting thought. You are much more than that. Don't let the past define who you are. You are greater than your past.

Imagine you are driving a boat on a beautiful calm lake. You look into the water behind your boat and you see the wake. This tells you where you have been, but not where you are going! *You* are driving your boat of life and *you* decide where you are going. With anxiety and/or depression, the steering wheel or helm gets locked into a sharp turn and the boat swings around and catches up with its own wake (past) and there is no more direction, just a downward spiral. Take back control by ignoring the dead past and drive your boat towards your goals. If you get a distressing thought, create a new habit. Stop and ask yourself if that thought is coming from the dead, negative past. If the answer is 'yes', just let it go! You are not dead; you are not negative—you are positive; you are present!

Use the magic four-letter word (and it's not what you may think!): STOP. This four-letter word stops everything. When you have an upsetting thought, test it. Say, 'STOP!' Then ask, 'What exactly is that thought?' The moment you have asked that question, you have become the observer, so you are already not in the thought— you are identifying it and therefore observing it, so, already, you are well on the way to freeing yourself from it. Then ask yourself if there is any evidence to support that thought. In the vast majority of cases, you will see that there is no evidence. For example, if it's a 'what if', 'perhaps', or 'maybe' type of thought, there is no evidence. Anxiety makes everything that's uncertain seem certain.

Occasionally the 'what if' thought can have some validity. If that happens, use the 'if... then...' technique. In other words, have a plan. For example, '*If* it rains tomorrow, *then* I'll postpone my gardening plans and catch up on my reading.' When we have a plan, it greatly reduces anxiety.

If it's an 'if only' type of thought, it is dead, because it is in the past and the past cannot be changed. Remember—if it has happened in the past, that is no evidence that it will happen in the future. If there is no evidence, or the thought is dead, just let that thought go! If the thought is fact, then we are better equipped to deal with it because it is real. Anxiety is most often caused when we believe things that are not real, and dealing with something that is not real is impossible and, therefore, self-destructive. Keep practising these techniques and, like driving your car, new ways of thinking will become automatic.

# 5. Don't try to do the impossible—you are not perfect.

Perfectionism is related to depression because the perfectionist can never be satisfied and can never know that feeling of contentment, which is a key to happiness. If a perfectionist achieves a goal, it is not enough. Having done something perfectly, the perfectionist invariably thinks it could have been done even more perfectly! If the perfectionist falls just short of the goal, the despair arising from self-flagellation creeps in. If the goal is not even attempted because the perfectionist believes the goal is beyond their capabilities, this misery can easily metamorphosise into depression. Perfectionists become more and more self-analytical and self-critical as they get older.

If you are a perfectionist, you have self-limiting thoughts, so use the STOP techniques.

*'STOP! What is that thought?'*

- Answer: 'I won't be able to get 100% for this maths exam.'
- Question: 'Am I looking inward or outward?'
- Answer: 'Inwards.'
- Statement: 'Looking inward is making me a victim. Victims end up with depression.'
- Answer: 'I'm going to look outward and let that thought go.'

*'STOP! What is that thought?'*

- Answer: 'I won't be able to get 100% for this maths exam.'
- Question: 'Do I have any evidence for that thought?'

- Answer: 'No.'
- Statement: 'If there is no evidence, let that thought go.'

*'STOP! What is that thought?'*

- Question: 'But what if I don't get 100%?'
- Answer: 'Deal with it if and when it becomes a fact.'
- Question: 'But I know I'll feel terrible if I don't. What then?'
- Answer: 'No facts—so let it go.'

If the perfectionist falls short of the goal and gets 95%, again apply the above techniques:

*'STOP! What is that thought?'*

- Answer: 'I feel terrible, I only got 95%.'
- Question: 'Are you looking inward or outward?'
- Answer: 'Inward.'
- Statement: 'You are playing the victim and heading for depression.'
- Response: 'I'm going to drop that thought.'

*Reframe!* Is there *another way* you can look at your result of 95%? By reframing, we can move from worrying about 5% to celebrating 95%. One is negative, and the other is positive. One heals, the other destroys. It's our choice. Practise, practise, practise! Remember—no-one is perfect, including ourselves!

# 6. Just accept and smile!

Just accept what you can't change. The most important part of happiness is contentment. You could be the busiest person in the world and be content, or you could be sitting on your backside and be content. It's that feeling that everything is going along nicely. The road to contentment is acceptance. It's that wonderful feeling that comes, for example, from just accepting that we love someone, despite their limitations, and accepting that we too have our limitations.

You don't have to buy into the games that people play if you don't like them. In Shakespeare's brilliant monologue from his play, *As You Like It*, Jaques (one of the characters) says:

'All the world's a stage and all the men and women merely players.'

So it is with life. Each person is playing a role—and so are we. For instance, there's the victim, the Good Samaritan, the manipulator, the curmudgeon, the chatterbox, the emotional blackmailer, the clown, the controller, the narcissist, the sociopath, the crowd pleaser, and so on. Once we can identify the role or game, we have a choice—do we buy in or don't we? If we can use our powers of acceptance and allow people to do what they do and play the games they play, we can be unaffected by these games and roles. We just accept that it's their game and we don't have to be a part of it unless we want to.

It is also important to be realistic and non-judgemental in our assessment of others and their games. This technique also gives us the ability to look at our own part on the stage of life. What's our role? If we like it, that's fine. If we don't, we have a choice. We can either accept it and learn to love it, or we can change the game by changing the habits and behaviours we don't like.

Stop seeking the approval of others and start accepting yourself—warts and all! Appreciate the good things about yourself. Loving yourself is the most important love you can have because, after all, if you don't love yourself, you can't expect others to love you. It's nice to be loved, so start with yourself! None of us is perfect and by accepting and even loving our imperfections (because that's who we are), we change our vibrations and attract new friends, relationships and opportunities.

And SMILE! Do the toothpaste drill. When you go to the bathroom and reach for the toothpaste, look into the mirror and smile at your reflection. Even though you may not feel like smiling, make yourself smile. You will instantly trigger a positive brain response and feel a lot happier than before you smiled. The act of smiling spurs a reaction in the brain, releasing certain hormones, including dopamine (also a neurotransmitter), which increases our feelings of happiness. In addition, your reflection is smiling back at you! Smile at as many people as possible during your day, and you will be amazed at how many people return the smile as this continues to lift your mood—and theirs!

# 7. Avoid jumping to conclusions.

It is important to look at things from a different perspective—
we can't change what has happened to us, but we can change
the way we look at it. We all look at things differently, based on
our learnt programs. Take a simple example of a plus sign. A
religious person might see it as representing the cross on which
Jesus was crucified. A practical person might see it as a positive
sign on a battery terminal. Another might see it as an arithmetical
plus sign and so on. Our memories of the past are also coloured
by our ingrained programs. We must create the habit of stopping
and asking ourselves if there is another way to view what has
happened because jumping to conclusions can be dangerous to
our mental health.

Take the example of an unreturned phone call.

> 'She hasn't called me back because she doesn't care! I feel so
> angry after all I have done for her.'

This is jumping to conclusions. She could have misplaced her
phone. Her battery could have gone flat. She might have had
urgent business. She might have been extremely busy, and it
slipped her mind. It is important to recognise other possibilities.
It's okay to say, 'I don't know why she didn't call me back,' and let
it go without attributing sinister scenarios.

Another good habit to practise is looking at the possible intention
behind a comment or deed, rather than the action itself. Often
people say something quite innocently, but we pick on a word or
image used, connect it to something from our past (via our trigger
points) and allow ourselves to be angry, hurt or offended. Taking

a moment to think about the possible intention behind what was said before we react can free us from so much hurt.

It is essential to cultivate the habit of seeing things from different perspectives. Remember—the way we interpret things determines our mood.

So, look at the glasses through which you are seeing the world around you. *What kind of glasses are you wearing?* For instance:

- Are you looking at the world through fear glasses? Is everything scary and dangerous?
- Are you looking through shitty glasses? Is everything turning to shit?
- Are you looking through dark glasses that view everything based on past experience? (Remember, if it has happened in the past, it is not evidence that it will happen in the future.)

If your glasses are negative, take them off by recognising what they are, and put on your positive or happy glasses and you will see the world differently!

## 8. Goal setting—take small steps towards your goal.

Decide on your goals and get motivated! What's stopping you? Depression often causes poor motivation and decision-making and this in turn often leads to deeper depression. Depression causes itself! Global thinking is what makes issues seem so big that they can't be handled—it is what leads us to feel overwhelmed and paralysed into inaction. Examples of these thoughts are: 'I just want to be happy,' and, 'I just want to feel normal.' Global thinking is a major cause of poor motivation and depression because things we want seem so huge, remote and unachievable. This in turn makes it hard for us to focus and get started. The renowned American actor and writer Sanford Meisner (1905–1997) said:

'That which hinders your task is your task.'

We fight global thinking by seeing what we want as a specified goal with its obstacles (rather than an unrealistic dream) and focusing on what we can do today towards that goal.

For example, take the thought, 'I just want to be happy.' Specify what you mean by happy, then ask yourself:

'What can I do right now? For a start I will live in the present moment and make myself smile. Then I will go for a walk or a run, visit a positive, happy friend, watch a comedy, go to a movie, or get into the car and go for a drive.'

By doing these sorts of things, we move closer to our goal of being happy instead of seeing it as a distant, paralysing, overwhelming and impossible dream and therefore taking no action. In extreme cases, the simple act (for example) of having a shower seems overwhelming. It becomes possible when we take that shower in small steps, focusing on each step, rather than on the end result. For example, check to see that we have what we need in the shower—soap, shampoo, towel, etc., then check that we have clothes ready to put on after the shower and so on. These are small steps, but focusing on each one leads steadily to the end result. We can easily become overwhelmed by the feeling that it will be impossible to reach our goals, and this makes us demotivated. Our goals should be achievable, not unrealistic.

We should also consider if it is really what we want. For instance, a goal of earning more money may not be what we really want. People who choose time and experiences over money and possessions are generally happier. The results of a study led by Dr Hal Hershfield from the University of California were published in May 2016. Below is an extract from the findings.

> Money and time are both scarce resources that people believe would bring them greater happiness. But would people prefer having more money or more time? And how does one's preference between those resources relate to happiness? Across studies, we asked thousands of Americans whether they would prefer more money or more time. Although the majority of people chose more money, choosing more time was associated with greater happiness.

The psychology department at Yale University, in a large-scale experience-sampling study, found that consumers derived value from anticipation and that value tended to be greater for experiential than for material purchases. We derive greater happiness from the anticipation of experiential purchases (for example, travel) than from material purchases (for example, a car, a boat, etc.). In other words, waiting for an experience tends to be more pleasurable and exciting than waiting to receive a material possession.

So, people who choose time and experiences (doing things) over money and material possessions tend to be happier. A brand-new expensive car might bring initial happiness, but a year later that joy is far less. An overseas holiday will bring the same joy a year later when savoured in our memories.

Once we have set a goal, it is important to specify that goal. For example, if the goal is to be able to meditate, specify what you mean. How long do I want to be able to meditate in a session? How many times per week? What time or times of the day? What is standing in my way (obstacles)? Specificity makes the goal real. Then focus on the steps leading to the goal and the steps to deal with any real obstacles which may impede. (This is the 'If... then...' approach. '*If* this happens, *then* I'll do that'). What can I do today to take a step towards my goal? As we take each step, the goal gets closer and feels more achievable.

In 1999, Dr Pham and Dr Taylor from the University of California conducted an experimental study with undergraduate students studying for their first mid-term examination in introductory psychology, where they compared process simulation (looking at the steps towards achieving the goal, including obstacles) and outcome simulations (simply visualising the final goal.)[17] Participants who were instructed to visualise themselves studying for the exam began studying earlier, spent more hours studying and performed better on the exam than participants instructed to

---

17 Pham, L. B., & Taylor, S. E. (1999). *From thought to action: Effects of process-versus outcome-based mental simulations on performance.* Personality and Social Psychology Bulletin, 25, 250-260.

imagine themselves attaining a high score on the exam. Process simulations reduced anxiety and facilitated planning.

Here is an extract from the study:

A widely held belief, particularly among members of the lay public, is that thinking positively about the future motivates self-regulated behaviour change in the present: 'If you dream it, you can achieve it.' The current study suggests that, on the contrary, it is more effective to mentally contrast positive thoughts about a desired future with obstacles standing in its way. Wishful thinking is, alas, exactly that. Anticipating enjoyment of achieving future goals feels good in the moment but has been shown in longitudinal studies to predict greater distress, dissatisfaction, and dysfunction. Less eloquent but more helpful advice for children would be — 'If you dream it, you have just begun.' Now consider the obstacles standing in the way of achieving your dream. Make and follow a plan to get around these obstacles. You will in this way help your dream come true.

Another very useful tool for goal setting is the WOOP method postulated by Dr Gabriele Oettingen in her book, *Rethinking Positive Thinking: Inside the New Science of Motivation.* You will notice that she includes obstacles. In some ways this contradicts Napoleon Hill's bestseller, *Think and Grow Rich* and to a lesser degree, Norman Vincent Peal's classic *The Power of Positive Thinking.*

**W** – what is my goal (my **W**ish)?

**O** – the best **O**utcome

**O** – potential **O**bstacles

**P** – if... then... **P**lan

Let's again use the example of meditation—this time with WOOP.

*Wish*      I would like to be able to meditate.

*Outcome*    I will be content, relaxed, focused, motivated, more intelligent, confident, and more socially connected.

*Obstacles*   Finding the time, finding the place, remembering to do it.

*Plan*      This is where the 'If..then...' plan comes in. You make a plan to deal with the obstacles. For instance: '*If* I forget to meditate, *then* I will do it before I go to bed.'

'The solution isn't to do away with dreaming and positive thinking. Rather, it's making the most of our fantasies by brushing them up against the very thing most of us are taught to ignore or diminish — the obstacles that stand in our way.'[18]

---

18 Gabrielle Oettingen, *Rethinking Positive Thinking*, 2015

# 9. Avoid disconnecting habits.

As we saw in Part 1, relationship issues repeatedly cause depression and disconnecting habits. What are these disconnecting habits? The seven most common are:

- Blaming
- Criticising
- Complaining
- Threatening
- Nagging
- Rewarding to gain control
- Punishing.

If the list above are the seven most common habits of disconnection, what are the seven most common connecting habits? These are:

- Encouraging
- Listening
- Supporting
- Trusting
- Respecting
- Accepting
- Negotiating differences.

It's a good idea to copy the two lists above and stick them onto your fridge door as a daily reminder to practise the connecting habits and avoid the disconnecting ones. The above lists are inspired by William Glasser, author of the best-selling book, *Choice Theory*.

*Below are two examples of relationship disconnection.*

In her collection of fascinating essays titled *Coventry*, award-winning Canadian-born British writer Rachel Cusk examines the disconnection in her early life. In the essay of the same title, she recounts how her parents would punish her with long periods of silence ('Coventry') and how they sent her to a boarding school for seven years and that boarding school was within walking distance from her home! If we examine her life, that learnt program of disconnection runs through it, in relationships —personally, socially and professionally—and also within the pettifoggery of some in the literary world.

Award-winning Jewish Hungarian-born (and later Canadian) physician, writer and speaker, Dr Gabor Maté describes how in 1945, towards the end of World War II during the German occupation of Hungary and extermination of Jews, his mother gave him to a stranger at the age of one in order to protect him from the Nazis. He was returned to his mother a month later, when Hungary was liberated, but Maté maintained that he was too young to understand why his mother had done this. He interpreted it as disconnection and abandonment and not being wanted. He maintains that he compensated by withdrawing within himself and having a great need to be needed. He was diagnosed with ADD. In his need to be wanted, he eventually turned to medicine and struggled very hard to pass his exams because of an inability to concentrate, caused by his ADD. Medical practice satisfied his desire to be wanted as he worked tirelessly to help his patients. Ironically, this caused his family to suffer as they in turn became disconnected from him.[19]

The choice is ours—so let's choose to start connecting! Let's break the disconnecting program by practising new habits. Start engaging with positive people, groups, hobbies, associations, etc. If you are lonely and like animals, get a dog, a cat or even a bird. We can learn so much from dogs. They give us unconditional love and loyalty, and they make us go out for walks!

---

19 Gabor Maté's publications are worth reading. One of his most fascinating books is *When the Body Says No: The Cost of Hidden Stress*. You will find some of his interviews and talks on YouTube.

# 10. Step outside your comfort zone.

Challenge yourself! Make a regular practice of doing something that you would normally regard as too hard, challenging or scary. When we do this, we build self-esteem, and self-esteem is a powerful antidote to both anxiety and depression. Have you heard people say, 'Take care,' as you're about to leave? Think about that for a moment. The message implies that there is danger out there and we should take care. My mother used to say, 'Take risks,' and that was one of her many wise sayings that I have adopted, but with one small addition—I say, 'Take risks—except when you're driving!'

Avoiding stepping out of our comfort zones can result in extreme social anxiety, where we find people whose world has shrunk through fear. For example, some people spend most of the day in a self-imposed prison—the bedroom—where they spend their lives playing internet games with virtual people. Connection and relationships with real people are vital to our mental health, but these people are connecting with virtual people through games with others who are invariably trapped in their own confined environment. This is the *connection of disconnection*. Their world has shrunk into their bedrooms, and they are fearful of the real world. In severe cases, they are scared to apply for work, to drive a car, to go into a shop or to accept an invitation to a party. Tragically, this usually ends in severe depression.

The way out for these people is to take even the tiniest step and then gradually build on this with activities such as fetching the mail from the mailbox. The next step could be walking 100 metres along the road in front of the house, then 200 metres, then walking to a shop or post office, then buying a stamp (having to talk to a stranger). Another approach is to undertake an activity and ask, 'What is my anxiety level now?' Maybe the answer is 10. Do the identical activity the next day and ask the same question. The answer will be less—say, 8. This technique is known as desensitisation and the more we repeat an action, the more we become desensitised. These small building blocks grow and lead us out of our ever-shrinking, self-imposed prisons of the mind.

# 11. Become socially connected.

Our social connections matter. Research shows that happy people spend more time with others and have a richer set of social connections than unhappy people. Studies even show that the simple act of talking to a stranger on the street can boost our mood more than we expect.

Try to focus on making one new social connection per day. It can be a short one or two-minute chat—such as sparking a conversation with someone on the train, asking a colleague or co-worker about their day, or even chatting to the barista at a coffee shop. But you should seek out more meaningful social connections, too. At least once this week, take a whole hour to connect with someone you care about—a friend who is far away or a family member you haven't talked to in a while. The key is that you must take the time needed to genuinely connect with another person.

Try to associate with happy people. When we are surrounded by positivity, it can easily rub off onto us. Similarly, when we associate with negative people and those that see themselves as victims, this also rubs off.

With the advent of COVID-19 and lockdowns and through no fault of their own, people have become socially isolated and micromanaged, seeing themselves as victims through incessant media negativity and fearmongering. This is a major contribution to the dramatic growth in anxiety and depression, So, avoid watching the harmful hypnotic repetition of the news and commentary, needles in arms, the negativity of radio shock jocks, etc. If there is something you need to know, you can rest assured that someone will tell you! Play music that you enjoy—watch inspiring TV shows and listen to uplifting podcasts. Connect for at least an hour a day with a friend far away and exercise as much as possible—ideally with a friend.

If you are working from home, try to work in a room with plenty of natural light and if possible, a pleasant view. Make sure that your workstation has an ergonomically comfortable chair and that your computer is the correct height for good posture. Take regular breaks from the screen and break up the day by doing things like calling a friend, making a cup of tea, or taking short walks.

# 12. Set aside a time to worry.

Make time to worry! Set aside an hour or half an hour at the same time each day—that is going to be your special time to worry! Then, during the day or night, whenever you get a stressful or anxious thought, pop it into your worry jar or pigeonhole and tell yourself that you will deal with it during your next worry hour. When whatever time you have chosen to worry comes, settle down—maybe with a cup of tea—and say, 'Now I'm ready to worry.' Open your worry jar and you will find that most of the power has gone from whatever you were planning to worry about. You may not even remember most of those worries. Even if, in the highly unlikely event that you do find an hour of worries, it's better than a whole day of worrying!

# 13. Get quality sleep.

Dr D.F. Dinges and Dr J.S. Durner from the University of Pennsylvania conducted a very interesting sleep study in 2005. They deprived one group of subjects of sleep (4.98 hours) and compared them with another group who were allowed normal sleep (7.4 hours). This and other similar studies repeatedly showed that lack of sleep had a negative impact on mood, memory, cognitive performance (ability to learn), motor function and physical health. This has huge implications for safety in the workplace—from surgeons to transport and the operation of heavy machinery.[20]

A famous study by Dr U. Wagner (2004) from the University of Lübeck in Germany revealed that sleep improves insight and creativity.[21]

*Normal sleep makes us happier.*

We all know what happens when a child has a sleepless night—adults are not much different! We wake up tired, emotional, unmotivated, and irritable, and often with a sense of pointlessness. In most cases of insomnia, it is our thoughts that keep us awake. These thoughts frequently come from anxiety-driven hypervigilance.

---

20 See under References at the end of this book for a comparative study on working hours regulations related to fatigue in the transport industry.

21 See under References at the end of this book for more information on this study.

Here are some non-drug techniques to deal with those thoughts.

- Go to bed before 10 pm, and don't work, exercise, watch television or play with electronic devices for at least an hour before going to bed.

- Don't go to bed straight after a big meal. Try to leave at least two hours between eating and going to bed. (Digesting a main meal can cause sleeplessness—not to mention weight gain!)

- Use distraction—if we try to fight our thoughts, we usually lose. A useful technique is to distract the mind by giving it something unimportant to think about. While the mind is preoccupied with this task, the thoughts that keep us awake fade away and we sleep. For example: We could think of four countries, cities, towns or villages beginning with the letter A, and then B and so on. Usually, by the time we get to around the letter K, we have fallen asleep. The next night it could be movies, actors, books, TV shows; and the next, the names of girls, then boys and so on.

- Get on the front foot—instead of fighting the thoughts, invite them in. Say to yourself, 'I want a thought right now. Come on thought... I want you right now.' Keep on inviting a thought, and you will most likely find that a thought doesn't come! If one does, say to yourself, 'Thank you—I'll just pop that thought into my thought jar and deal with it during my worry hour tomorrow. Now, come on, I want another thought right now.' It usually won't come!

- Breathe in to the count of four, hold the breath to the count of seven and then exhale to the count of eight. Do this five times. If you forget how many times you have done it, you must start again. This technique works because it is a highly relaxing breathing ratio which also requires some concentration, thus distracting the mind from irritating and disturbing thoughts and allowing relaxation-induced quality sleep.

- Listen to sleep meditations by people like Deepak Chopra, Eckhart Tolle and Sadhguru.[22]

- Repeat the mental mantra, 'I have no thoughts,' with each inhaled breath and, 'My thoughts have gone,' with each exhaled breath. If a thought pops up, say to yourself, 'That's a thought, but I have no thoughts,' and let it go. Notice that the gaps between the thoughts get longer, and then you sleep. Occasionally, a particularly invasive thought might slip in and you find yourself following it and other thoughts linked to it. Stop and tell yourself that it's just another thought, but that your mind is clear, so let it go. The repetition of the mantra makes the letting go much easier. Another effective way is to say on each outgoing breath, 'One, no thoughts, two, no thoughts, three, no thoughts,' and so on, with the aim of getting to 50 without a thought. Stop and go back if a thought sneaks in. You will usually be asleep long before 50!

- Try progressive muscle relaxation. It is described in strategy number 30.

---

22 See under References at the end of the book for Chopra, Tolle and Sadhguru sleep meditations.

# 14. Become the observer and healer—not the victim.

Observing ourselves in an emotion is much better than being in that emotion—it's a good starting point. Here is an effective way to do this.

1. If you experience an unwanted emotion, say 'STOP!' Then distance yourself from that emotion by becoming the observer and asking yourself, *'What emotion am I experiencing?'* By giving it a label, you are already the observer, not the participant. Your answer could be for example, 'sadness'.

2. Then ask yourself, *'Am I allowed to experience sadness?'* Yes, of course I am! There is no law against feeling sad. You have now removed the guilt which so often accompanies negative emotions.

3. Next, ask yourself, *'Will it last?'* No, it won't. Nothing on this earth lasts. You have now created the possibility of change.

4. Then ask, *'Do I want to remain a victim of sadness?'* No, I don't. You are now giving yourself a choice.

5. Now ask, *'Can I stop?'* Yes! You are now making that choice.

6. Finally ask, *'When?'* NOW. You have now taken action!

# 15. Mindfulness, meditation and hypnosis.

In a paper published by Harvard psychologists Matthew Killingsworth and Daniel Gilbert in 2010, they found that 46% of the time, we are not thinking about what we should be focused on. Our brain switches to our default network when not focused and wanders towards something most often driven by our underlying programs from the past. Mind-wandering can push us towards unhappiness. If, instead, we are thinking of (or focused on) what we are doing or good memories or positives, that's good. If we let our minds wander, then most of the time it's not good.[23]

Meditation is an excellent antidote as it takes the mind away from wandering, gives us focus and, with practice, creates a new inner peace and therefore a new way of thinking. In research conducted by Britta K Hölzel from the Harvard Medical School et al. in 2011, it was proved that meditation actually increases happiness and even IQ![24]

## How to meditate

Meditation is not hard to do if you are patient. Here is one simple approach.

1. Find comfortable place to sit.

   A place that feels safe, peaceful quiet and calm to you.

---

23 For more information about this paper, see under References at the end of this book *A wandering Mind is an Unhappy Mind.*

24 For more information about this paper, see under References at the end of this book *Mindfulness practice leads to increases in regional brain grey matter density.*

2. Set a time limit.

   If you're just beginning, choose a short time—like 5 or 10 minutes.

3. Choose a position you can stay in.

   You can sit in a chair with your feet on the floor or sit cross-legged. (Many experienced meditators feel comfortable in the lotus position). You can kneel if you prefer. Any position is okay as long as you are stable and in a position you can maintain.

4. Become aware of your body.

   With your eyes closed, or open, just notice the parts of your body—scalp, face, neck and shoulders, etc.

5. Feel your breath.

   Now focus on your breathing and observe the sensation of your breath as it goes in and as it goes out.

6. Notice when your mind has wandered.

   Your attention will leave the focus on your breath and wander to other places. When you notice that your mind has wandered, don't be angry—be kind to yourself and simply return your attention to the breath and keep on doing this each time your mind wanders.

7. Close with kindness.

   When you're ready, gently open your eyes, or lift your gaze if they are open. Take a moment and notice any sounds in the environment. Notice how your body is feeling and observe your thoughts and emotions.

That's basically all there is to it. This method might not suit you, so there are many forms of meditation. Here are some of them.

- mindfulness meditation
- spiritual meditation
- focused meditation
- movement meditation
- mantra meditation
- transcendental meditation
- progressive relaxation
- loving-kindness meditation.

There are many inexpensive classes and groups that will help you to learn the techniques of mindfulness and/or meditation. These techniques give us a sense of inner peace and calm, which results in a more positive outlook. They empower us and help us to focus and acquire new skills in self-management. It's a good idea to find meditation clips and podcasts from people like Sadhguru, Maharishi Mahesh Yogi, Deepak Chopra and Eckhart Tolle— there are plenty more.[25]

Hypnosis helps us to dump the baggage from the past and to heal. Find a good clinical hypnotherapist or learn the techniques of self-hypnosis.

---

25 At the end of this book under References, you will see links to some of these people.

# 16. Hypnotise yourself and build expectancy.

Your subconscious mind never sleeps. It has been awake 24/7 since you were born. When you wake up in the morning, your subconscious mind is still fully awake and dominant. So, you have a clear 30-second window of opportunity to put something directly into your own subconscious mind from your conscious mind while it is still waking up. If your first thought is, for example, 'I'm going to have a calm day,' that unfiltered, unmodified message goes straight into your subconscious and you will be amazed at how calm your day will be! Building expectancy is important—things can and will change. Be open to change or the possibility of it.

# 17. A word about addiction.

As we saw in Part 1, addiction is often the result of a well-intentioned, but misguided attempt by the conscious mind to reduce or eliminate the pain of a subconscious program emanating from past (usually childhood) experiences. For example, alcohol or drugs are adopted in an attempt to block emotional pain and food is adopted for comfort.

Alcohol and drugs are recognised depressants and a cause of anxiety, especially when excessively consumed. We may feel great when we're drunk—full of confidence and the life and soul of the party. However, it is the next day and the days following that bring on the anxiety and depression. A large proportion of alcoholics and drug users started off by being shy teenagers. Alcohol and drugs suddenly gave them a feeling of confidence, so they went on with it—too often and too much.

Alcohol is a drug, but, in our culture, it has become accepted as essential for most social gatherings. Perhaps we should drink for the taste and not for the effect! There is far more alcohol-induced than illicit drug-induced violence in Australia. According to a report from the US National Institute on Alcohol Abuse and Alcoholism published on February 16, 2018, drinking is considered to be in the moderate or low-risk range for women at no more than three drinks in any one day and no more than seven drinks per week. For men, it is no more than four drinks a day and no more than 14 drinks per week.

Peer group pressure to binge-drink and use illicit drugs is enormous in young people, and it is one of the reasons why we have become an anxious country. It is important to seek help if you feel that you *have to* have a drink, or smoke weed, or use speed, meth, etc. It is heartbreaking to see so many young lives being wasted through addiction.

Levels of addiction have grown at a frightening rate in Australia. Gambling is an example of this, as we have the highest pro-rata rate of gambling in the world, with $24 billion being lost per annum. (The largest losses come from the pokies, followed by casinos and then the TAB.)

A major cause of substance addition is the over-prescription of opioids. The Australian Institute of Health and Welfare, an independent statutory Australian Government Agency reports that in 2016–2017, 15.4 million opioid prescriptions were dispensed under the Pharmaceutical Benefits Scheme. During this period, 40,000 people used heroin, while 715,000 people used pain-killing opioids (mostly oxycodone) for illicit or non-medical purposes. Legal or pharmaceutical opioids are responsible for more deaths and hospitalisations than illegal opioids such as heroin. In 2016 deaths from pharmaceutical opioid misuse accounted for 62% of all drug-induced deaths.

While there is not much we as individuals can do about this shocking rate of over-prescription, it is important that we encourage others and ourselves to consider other ways to control pain, such as hypnosis, acupuncture, myotherapy, Bowen Therapy, osteopathy, meditation, yoga and many more. If we feel we cannot do without pain medication, we should request non-opioid analgaesics.

We often hide behind the word 'addicted' because it gives us a convenient excuse and implies that there is nothing we can do about it. *This is not so!* Addiction is a habit, and a habit is a behaviour. Everyone has choice. We can always change a behaviour *if we choose to*, and, similarly, as we know from the strategies in this section, it's about changing the way we think.

'STOP!' What am I about to do? Write the word STOP! on the back of your hand so you read it when you reach for a cigarette, a drink, a piece of cake, a joint, a pipe or your TAB account on your phone!

There are a number of government-funded, privately funded and charity organisations that work in the area of addiction. Some of these are AIVL, ANEX, ADF, HRA, Family Drug Support Australia, Gamblers Help, ReachOut Australia and so on.

I do a lot of work with people who have various addictions and have found that hypnosis is a powerful tool. A good way to find a suitable hypnotherapist is to search through the directories of hypnotherapy associations like the AHA, AACHP and the HCA. In order to belong to an association, the therapist has to possess government-accredited qualifications.

# 18. Let go of your guilt.

Guilt comes from the past. What we have done, we have done —that can't be changed. However, it is healing to apologise, then make amends if we can and learn from the experience. It is important to make sure that the apology is sincere and unconditional (without excuses). It is irrelevant whether the person accepts the apology or not—it is the act of apologising that is liberating. We are imperfect and we are wired for struggle, but *we are worthy of love and belonging.* We must be to be able to say we're sorry and will fix it instead of passing the blame on. If it is not possible to apologise (for instance, if the person is no longer alive or contactable), then what has been done has been done— nothing can change that, so learn from it, let it go, and move on.

We should have the courage to admit our imperfections and not be afraid to fail. (Blame is an unhealthy and ineffective way to discharge guilt, pain and discomfort.) Once we have done these things, we must let it go and move on. To let the dead past control us is a recipe for disaster. Carrying guilt is an unnecessary, negative, and emotionally harmful burden. We must be sure to avoid excessive and unfounded guilt, as we are only punishing ourselves and no-one else. So, 'STOP!' and let those 'if only' thoughts go.

The more you allow guilt to make you critical of yourself the more you damage yourself.

- You can't change the past. You've made really stupid decisions, but those decisions no longer matter because they are in the past.
- By constantly examining yourself, living in the dead past

and criticising yourself, you become the victim and victims never get better.

- Take charge of your life. Stop being self-centred and focusing on you and your needs and your troubles.
- Look out at the world outside you and see the positives.
- Take off your dark negative glasses and put on your bright sunshine glasses.
- Once you do this, you will see the good and not just the bad.

You become a new person. People forgive you and start to like you again. You are the only person who can do this. Don't forget you always have a choice. As soon as you think you don't have a choice, you are once again playing the victim.

# 19. Avoid uncertainty.

Uncertainty and indecision are the food of anxiety, and anxiety is the food of depression. Being unable to make up our minds about something can lead to anxiety and on to depression. As Marie Beynon Ray wrote in her book, *How to Conquer your Handicaps*:

> Indecision is fatal. It is better to make a wrong decision than build up a habit of indecision. If you're wallowing in indecision, you certainly can't act—and action is the basis of success.

*So, even a bad decision can be better than no decision!*

Deal with facts—they are easier to handle than fiction. Avoid uncertainty by making an effort to find out. Take, for example, someone who has had an inconclusive, or (even worse) no diagnosis of a troubling medical condition and therefore no prognosis. Rather than slide into anxiety and depression through agonising about what it could be, that person should get a second or third opinion— even more if necessary. Once we have a proper diagnosis (even if it's a bad one), we feel so much better simply because we know what we're dealing with. If we only dealt with facts, our anxiety would be under control.

# 20. Imagine your perfect day.

Write down your perfect day using your imagination. It could be at home, or on a tropical island in Tahiti—anywhere your imagination takes you. Describe everything you do on that perfect day from the time you wake up till the time you go to bed. Write it in the present tense, and when you describe each imagined event, write how you are feeling about the event (your emotions).

Imagination is an essential tool of hypnosis. Imagination is our gateway to the subconscious, and the subconscious is where our self-limiting programs are located. Read it each night before you go to sleep. By doing this you are using your imagination and using habituation, which is how we learn after the early years. Do this for two weeks and notice the change in your emotional state. Then, keep on with it at regular intervals and you will be surprised at how close you get to your perfect day because you have put those thoughts out there!

# 21. Don't fear change.

One of our greatest fears is change, and yet, one of the most certain things in the world is that things *will* change! Nothing stays the same. Even the particles in a rock are moving when examined under an electron microscope. We can't control change. Change is inevitable. So, by acknowledging that fact, we open ourselves to it and, in so doing, we become accepting—and acceptance is the pathway to contentment, and contentment is happiness! We must be open to change—or at least the possibility of change.

If we can't accept the inevitability of change, then we hurt ourselves. Take the example of people who fear ageing and can't accept the fact that their bodies are changing. Though ageing is inevitable, they can't accept this, so they make poor financial and health decisions and spend a fortune on plastic surgery—going through physical pain and trauma to buy a few years (at most) of admiration. 'Goodness! You are looking so young!' Often these people also have self-esteem issues, as they view themselves through what they think (but can't know) are the eyes of others.

*So, accept change because it is inevitable: don't fear it, and move on.*

# 22. Avoid mainstream and social media.

In Part 1, we looked at the staggering increase in anxiety and depression since the advent of social media. Mainstream media also has a lot to answer for. So much of what we are fed by the media is negative. 'Shock jocks' are a classic example. Not only do you have to listen to a self-important radio journalist pontificating, but the people who call in mostly do so to complain. Often people who listen to these shows have them playing in the background, which can be highly detrimental to establishing a positive, healthy state of mind. This is because our subconscious mind never sleeps and is aware of everything going on. And, being a computer, it accepts everything that's fed into it. Because the subconscious mind is running 90% of our day, these negative messages are not good. Many journalists have become activists, controlling the way they want us to see the news, rather than the news itself. They want us to be anxious and fearful, as this builds their audience—a newspaper focusing only on good news will always fail because fear is addictive.

Instead of watching or listening to this stuff, listen to your favourite music or an uplifting podcast. Reduce your time on social media platforms such as Facebook, Twitter, Snapchat etc. and avoid mainstream media and you will be amazed at the difference in your mood.

Duke Orsino in Shakespeare's comedy, *Twelfth Night,* says: *'If music be the food of love, play on!'* Love is a powerful antidote to anxiety and depression, so choose to listen to your favourite music. Play on and love!

# 23. What about grief?

It is important to allow ourselves to grieve. Grieving is natural and contributes to our recovery. However, when it becomes pervasive and starts to control our lives, it is time to rearrange our thought processes and deal with fact. We can deal with fact—it is what is *not real* that can truly hurt us.

So, it is a *fact* that a loved one has died. It is a *fact* that nothing can change that. Therefore, it is a *fact* that what we are doing, we are doing to ourselves and no-one else. It is also a *fact* that we have choice. It is a *fact* that we can choose to continue to hurt ourselves, and it is a *fact* that we can choose to stop!

Having dealt with these facts, we can move towards the positives. Would the person who we love and has died want us to suffer? If there is a spirit world and they are watching us, how would they be feeling watching someone they love indulging in self-torture? Would we like to honour their memory by living a good life and remembering the good things, or prefer to live in self-inflicted melancholy?

# 24. Stop being the judge and micromanager and let go of the need to control.

We only have control over ourselves. People are who they are—we can't change that, nor should we try. In attempting to change, control or micromanage others, we only frustrate ourselves and damage the recipients of our micromanagement. Once we accept this and learn to let go, we relieve ourselves of so much stress, frustration and anger.

Children who in those crucial pre-school years have been micromanaged frequently struggle with decision-making in later life. This leads to insecurity and is one reason why so many parents still have their children at home, well into their 20s and beyond!

Attempting to control what we can't control can cause damage to our emotional state. 'This is terrible weather.' It's not terrible weather—it's just weather and the 'terrible' part comes from us! 'This traffic is awful.' No—it's just traffic! When we try to control it, we become anxious, and because, in many cases, anxiety causes a fight response, this can result in behaviours like road rage. Remember, the ability to accept what we can't control is a highway to emotional freedom!

# 25. What about my work?

Anxiety and depression can often be increased by the work we do. We spend a large part of our lives at work—what can we do if we dislike the work we are doing or if our problem is workplace bullying? In both cases, we are wasting the most precious commodity we have—our time.

If we hate what we are doing, we not only waste a huge part of our lives, which we can never get back, but we also cause suffering to ourselves and our loved ones, who have to cope with our resultant bad moods. The solution is simple — change jobs. It's not just about money — our mental health is far more important.

People in jobs where they are not using their character strengths are less happy than those who are. In Martin Seligman's book, *Authentic Happiness*, he lists our character strengths and insists that the more of these you use in your job, the happier you will be. He says happiness is not the result of good genes or luck. Real, lasting happiness comes from focusing on one's personal strengths rather than weaknesses — and working with them to improve all aspects of one's life.

These character strengths (not in order of importance) are:

- Humour
- Bravery
- Self-regulation
- Curiosity
- Prudence
- Spirituality

- Open-mindedness
- Appreciation of beauty and excellence
- Love
- Gratitude
- Compassion
- Love of learning
- Creativity
- Forgiveness and mercy
- Fairness
- Social intelligence
- Integrity
- Citizenship
- Perspective
- Leadership
- Humility and modesty
- Vitality
- Hope
- Good judgement
- Zest

*Are you using your character strengths in your job? Change it if you are not!*

If our problem is not the work we do, but a workplace bully, below are some effective methods for dealing with that bully without getting upset or angry. If we get upset or angry, it's a victory for the bully. Instead, we can deal with that bully in a calm way, without raising our voice.

As an example: the bully says something hurtful to you. So, you respond with:

'I'm not sure I understood what you said—could you please repeat exactly the words you have just said to me?'

The bully then has to remember what he or she has just said. This requires rethinking, and usually the aggressor will say something like, 'What I meant to say was...' In other words, the bully has backed down and that is a win for you.

If the bully is self-opinionated, he or she might repeat exactly what they have just said. If that happens, you say:

'Thank you. I'm just going to write that down while it is fresh in my mind.'

The bully hates nothing more than being exposed as a workplace bully—a charge that can have serious ramifications not only for the bully, but also for the company or organisation. The bully might ask you why you are going to do that. Don't give an explanation—say it is your business, or it is personal.

You can also use a gentler strategy if the bully is being offensive with a rather personal comment. Simply say:

'How do you think that makes me feel?'

In order to answer your question, the bully has to put her or himself into your shoes. This usually results in a withdrawal. If the reply is, 'I don't care how you feel', then simply move to the strategy in the paragraph above.

# 26. Avoid words of control.

'I *must* get out of bed now. Then I *need to* have a shower because I *have to* have breakfast in time to catch the 8:00 train. I've *got to* be in time for the 9:00 staff meeting.'

Thoughts like these take the power away from us. Our subconscious mind simply accepts everything our conscious mind lets through. The message we are sending is that something is controlling us. We are using the words of control such as '*got to*', '*need to*', '*have to*', '*must*', '*ought to*', etc. We should avoid those words. Instead, think:

'*I'm getting* out of bed now, then *I'll have* a shower. After that *I'll have* breakfast because *I'm catching* the 8:00 train, so *I'll be* in time for the 9:00 staff meeting.'

You are now in control—there is nothing telling you that you 'need to', 'have to' and so on.

# 27. Take control over how much you eat and lift your self-esteem.

Weight issues are often caused by programs from our early years —for example, when we were told to eat everything on our plate and to think about the starving Africans. (I've never understood why eating everything on my plate helped the starving Africans!) This early program tells the subconscious that we have to eat when we are not hungry. In other words, this is overeating! Similarly, regular home and school mealtimes and tea breaks also add pressure to eat when not hungry. Because a child is vulnerable in those early years and because they mirror the behaviour of their parents without question, a parent who has poor eating habits unwittingly passes that behaviour on to the child, and that program sticks. This is often a cause of addiction to sweet things.

Diets tend not to work in the long-term because we are depriving ourselves of foods that the body craves—and eventually gets. It seems logical that if we continue to eat whatever we have been eating, but (for example) only two-thirds of it, our craving for foods denied in diets will be reduced because we are not depriving ourselves of them. The stomach will shrink, and we can reach a healthy weight. Sometimes it is a good tactic to take one-third of everything on your plate and put it into the waste bin. Better in the waste than on the waist! You will soon tire of this and just cook and eat less. And don't forget to masticate—the more you chew your food, the more your brain believes that you have eaten enough.

Temptation is a major issue with weight. So, change the situation and avoid temptation. For example, change visibility (proximity) by removing lollies or biscuits from the kitchen bench and replacing them with something healthy, like a bowl of fruit, for instance. Gertraud Stadler of Columbia University and Gabriele Oettingen of New York University undertook a study on this issue in 2014. Below are the results.

> There were main effects for both proximity and visibility. People ate an average of 2.2 more candies each day when they were visible and 1.8 candies more when they were proximately placed on their desk vs 2 metres away. It is important to note, however, that there was a significant tendency for participants to consistently underestimate their daily consumption of proximately placed candies and overestimate their daily consumption of less proximately placed candies. These results show that the proximity and visibility of a food can consistently increase an adult's consumption of it.

It is also a good idea to change the way we think about weight. People often come to me to 'lose weight'. I tell them I don't help people to lose weight. Instead, I help them to gain slimness. The first one is a negative, which also implies that you are losing something, so maybe you should get it back! The second is a positive aim. It's all about managing our thoughts and the way we view things.

I have been experimenting in ways to trick the brain. If you wear a mouth guard at night to stop grinding your teeth, keep wearing it as much as possible during the day within the constraints of social and work situations. It tricks the brain into believing that because you are biting on something, you are eating, and this can reduce your appetite and stop you snacking. It would probably work with a sports mouthguard too.

## 28. Manage your anger and anxiety by replay.

Consider the following scenario:

You are driving in the right lane just on the speed limit in heavy traffic and someone is tailgating you. You get angry and slow down to get up the nose of the tailgater. He gets angrier and starts flashing his lights and hooting. You get angrier and slow even more, holding up the traffic behind the tailgater. Your passenger becomes frightened and anxious. You are angry, your blood pressure is up, and the traffic behind you is becoming frustrated and angry.

Replay the scenario as follows:

You are driving in the right lane just on the speed limit in heavy traffic and someone is tailgating you. You feel irritated but realise that the only person over whom you have control is yourself. So you decide to move over to the left lane at the next opportunity. The tailgater flashes past and tailgates the next car in the right lane. You have accepted that he is what he is and let it go. Your passenger has noticed nothing and is calm and relaxed, and the drivers behind the tailgater are not frustrated with you.

There are four losers in the first scenario: the tailgater, you and your blood pressure, your passenger, and the drivers behind you.

There are four winners in the second scenario: you and your blood pressure, your passenger, the drivers behind you, and the increased chance that you will get safely to your destination! And who cares about the tailgater!

It is highly therapeutic to replay an incident where you have been angry and ask yourself if there is a better way that you could have handled the situation because you are more likely to stop yourself next time a similar situation occurs. The same applies if you have overreacted because of anxiety—replay what you have done in a different way and, next time a similar situation occurs, you will handle it differently.

## 29. Listen to your voice and to your speech habits.

The sound of someone's voice is often an indicator of their state of mind. For example, a whining, whingeing tone can be indicative of someone playing or being the victim or seeking pity and/or attention. A loud voice can indicate a controlling person or an extrovert demanding attention. (It can also be the voice of someone who is using a loud voice as a defence to cover up an underlying inferiority complex.) A well-modulated voice often indicates someone who is confident and balanced. A very soft voice can be an indication of someone who is insecure with low self-esteem. Many young adults (mostly female) still use a little child's voice when talking to older adults—usually indicating a subliminal need to be loved.

'STOP!' and listen to *your* voice. What game are you playing? Change the tone of your voice if it isn't indicating who you are or who you want to be. This will have a beneficial effect on your mental health.

Some of our speech habits can indicate features of our emotional states. These habits can indicate insecurity and therefore the need to know that we have attention and are being listened to.

Here are some examples:

- Repetition of the question, 'Right?'

  *'I went down the street, right? And there I saw a brand-new Bentley, right?'*

- Repetition of the words 'so yeah'. The word 'yeah' meaning 'yes' when needing reassurance—'Yes, you are with me.'

  *'I went to visit her in hospital, so, yeah. The doctor was just leaving, and I was lucky enough to be able to speak to him, so, yeah.'*

- Overuse of the words 'you know', again with the unconscious aim of needing to be supported.

  *'She's quite a good swimmer, you know, and, you know, I think, you know, she could end up in the Olympics one day, if, you know, she trains hard.'*

- The rising terminal—when we turn a normal sentence into what sounds like a question because our voice goes higher at the end of the sentence. Because it sounds like a question, it's a way of saying 'are you with me?'

  *'The other day Mark and I went to the races? There were some unruly people milling around, so I got this feeling that trouble was brewing?'*

Anxiety and depression impede clear thinking, so we often use padding to give us time to think. A typical example is the frequent repetition of the word 'like', which has become so common nowadays that there is no need for examples!

If you have any of these speech habits, start to change them. It will improve self-confidence and overall mental health.

# 30. Anti-freeze.

As we have seen earlier, there are three responses to anxiety—fight, flight and freeze. This exercise is about freeze—the emotions we have suppressed or pushed down. You might like to try one or both of the techniques that follow.

The first is an ancient, yoga-based technique which can help to reduce anxiety and PTSD symptoms, improve sleep and heal past emotional wounds. *If you have lower-back, hip or knee problems, don't try it.* Please read through to the last paragraph before you begin.

The second is designed to release physical pain frequently coming from suppressed emotions.

## Technique 1 — trembling for stress release.

1. Stretch out on your back on the floor, on a yoga mat or a carpet, or a firm bed and, if necessary, place a cushion or pillow under your head for comfort.

2. Keeping your feet on the ground, move your knees apart as widely as you can without discomfort and place the soles of your feet together so that the outside of each ankle is almost touching the floor.

3. Bring your feet up as close as you can to your bottom (keeping them on the floor). Do this without hurting yourself.

4. Now press down with your feet so that your hips lift up in the air. Lift them as high as you can, keeping your knees wide apart.

Hold that position until your legs start to tremble slightly due to muscular strain. (We are not talking about a swaying motion that your legs might develop. Ignore that—we are waiting for a trembling or slight shaking in the legs.)

5. Once that tremoring is felt, keeping the knees apart, slowly lower your hips until your bottom is on the ground.

6. When your bottom is on the ground with your knees wide apart, keep the soles of your feet together and very slowly start to move the knees closer together until they eventually touch.

7. On the way, you will probably find that your legs start to shake or tremble, even though there is no muscular strain. When this happens, keep those knees in that position until the trembling or shaking stops, and then continue to move those knees closer together until they shake again. Once again, keep them in that position until the shaking stops.

8. Keep on doing this until the knees eventually touch. This shaking may continue up through the stomach and chest and sometimes even through to the shoulders and up to the neck and head. (If your feet start to feel uncomfortable, it's okay to put them flat on the floor keeping the inner ankles together.)

In some cases, people might also feel emotional. Don't worry about that—they are good tears. They are tears of release, assisting in the release of tension stored in the body. If you concentrate on something that has upset you, you may find that the shaking increases. It is your tool, so apply it as you see fit.

If you don't experience the shaking, immediately repeat the process, but there is no need to repeat the hip lift. Stop when all trembling has stopped or when you feel tired—whichever comes first.

Repeat this exercise at least three times per week and you will be amazed at how much better you sleep and how much less anxious you are (having released the freeze part of your anxiety).

In some cases, the trembling doesn't happen. That might mean that you already let your emotions out and don't suppress them, or that you are subconsciously blocking. We block because there is a part of us that doesn't want to get better—because the anxiety is all we have ever known and the thought of change into the unknown world of calm is too much. Better the devil we know... If you block, it's okay. There are plenty of other strategies in this book that will help you to unblock.

## Technique 2 — Progressive Muscle Relaxation

Another technique is *Progressive Muscle Relaxation.*[26] Because the body is a mirror of the mind, when we feel anxious or stressed, this can be reflected in physical pain, for example, fibromyalgia. Have you ever had an aching back or pain in your neck when you were anxious or stressed? When you have anxiety or stress in your life, one of the ways your body responds is with muscle tension. Progressive Muscle Relaxation has been proved to be an effective method to relieve that tension and, in so doing, relieve physical pain.

In Progressive Muscle Relaxation, you tense a group of muscles as you breathe in, and you relax them as you breathe out. You work

26 Freeman L. *Relaxation therapy.* In Mosby's Complementary and Alternative Medicine: A Research-Based Approach, 3rd ed. 2009, pp. 129–157. St. Louis: Mosby Elsevier.

on your muscle groups in a certain order. When your body is physically relaxed, you're not anxious. The more you practise, the easier it gets.

When you first start, it may help to use an audio recording until you learn all the muscle groups in order. One such audio recording has been done by the *Newcastle upon Tyne Hospitals* and can be found on YouTube.[27]

*Technique 2—How you do it. (It's not the only way!)*

Choose a place where you can lie down on your back and stretch out comfortably, such as a carpeted floor or firm bed.

1. Breathe in and tense the first muscle group below (hard but not to the point of pain or cramping) for 5–10 seconds.
2. Breathe out, and suddenly and completely relax the muscle group (do not relax it gradually).
3. Relax for 10–20 seconds before you work on the next muscle group.
4. Notice the difference between how the muscles feel when they are tense and how they feel when they are relaxed.

When you have a very tense muscle, you can practise tensing and relaxing that muscle area without going through the whole routine.

---

27 Here is the link: https://youtu.be/912eRrbes2g
Here is another link to a YouTube audio recording—this one is by *Therapist Aid*: https://youtu.be/1nZEdqcGVzo

The following is a list of the muscle groups in order and how to tense them.

| Body part | Action |
|---|---|
| Hands | Clench them. |
| Wrists and forearms | Extend them and bend your hands back at the wrist. |
| Biceps and upper arms | Clench your hands into fists, bend your arms at the elbows, and flex your biceps. |
| Shoulders | Shrug them (raise toward your ears). |
| Forehead | Scrunch it into a deep frown. |
| The eyes and bridge of the nose | Close your eyes as tightly as you can. |
| Cheeks and jaws | Smile as widely as you can. |
| The lips | Press your lips together tightly. |
| Front of the neck | Touch your chin to your chest. |
| Back of the neck | Press the back of your head against the floor or bed. |

| Body part | Action |
| --- | --- |
| Chest | Take a deep breath and hold it for 5–10 seconds. |
| Back | Arch your back up and away from the floor or bed. |
| Stomach | Suck it into a tight knot. |
| Hips and buttocks | Press your buttocks together tightly. |
| Thighs | Clench them hard. |
| Lower limbs | Point your toes toward your face. Then point your toes away, and curl them downward at the same time. |

Take a nice deep breath and relax the mind. You will be amazed at how much less pain you are experiencing.

# 31. Dissociate yourself.

Hanging onto a painful experience is not good for your mental wellbeing. Here is a useful NLP-based technique to help free yourself from the control of a painful experience:

1. Close your eyes and take yourself into the feeling you have just had or are experiencing.

2. Feel it—feel the emotion and the pain till it gets to the maximum (around a 10 on a scale from 1 to 10). When you are in that place, imagine that you are stepping backwards, outside your body for a few paces and count those paces.

3. Stop and look at your body. Observe the painful expression and body language of you in that experience. Notice how your level of anxiety or emotional pain has become less since you have become the observer. It could, for example, be at level 8 or less.

4. Now, in your imagination, again step back, but this time take double the number of steps you first took. Now you are observing yourself looking at yourself in the experience. You have now become the observer of yourself observing yourself. Notice how your emotional pain has further diminished. Maybe it has gone down to a level 4 or lower.

5. Do this again—now you are observing yourself observing yourself observing yourself observing yourself in the experience! The experience has now become fourth-hand. You will notice that there is very little or no pain. If there is still some pain, repeat the process until you notice that the pain has gone.

6. Now pause and take your own lesson from this experience. Your lesson may be that you don't have to attach yourself to your anxiety, sadness or other emotion. Or it may be that you have a choice as to how you view your emotion. There could be many lessons.

7. Take your lesson, hold onto it, and now, in your imagination, go back through your stages of observation, thinking about the lesson until you are back in the place where you first experienced that pain. Apply your lesson and there will be no pain.

Practising this exercise will diminish future painful emotional experiences until they no longer trigger emotional pain and this exercise is no longer needed or you only need to step back once to release that emotion.

## 32. Talk to your inner child.

As mentioned earlier in the book, we all have an inner child. Think about your inner child and nurture her or him. When you are about to make a decision, pause and ask yourself, 'Is this good for my inner child?' If the answer is 'yes', then go ahead. If the answer is 'no', then take a different direction.

# 33. Cherish your experiences.

Cherishing is when we step outside of an experience to review and appreciate it. Often we fail to stay in the moment and really enjoy what we're experiencing. Cherishing intensifies and lengthens the positive emotions that come with doing something we love. For example, instead of thinking about a whole range of things while eating a delicious meal, cherish the sensations associated with eating—the taste, smell, texture, presentation and colours.

Pick one experience to truly cherish each day. It could be a nice shower, a delicious meal, a great walk outside, or any experience that you really enjoy. You may decide to share the positive experience with another person and think about how lucky you are to have enjoyed such an amazing moment. Sometimes it is a good idea to keep a personal souvenir or photo of that activity and make sure you stay in that present moment for the entire time you are looking at it. Each night, make a note of what you cherished.

# 34. Be kind.

I have always believed that in this world there are givers and takers. The givers are generous with their time and resources and experience happiness from the joy of sharing what they have received. The takers are parsimonious with time and resources and experience sadness from the fear of losing what they have taken.

Giving is more rewarding than receiving, so give smiles, say nice things and do kind things. Acts of kindness make us happier. Do kind things every day and your mood will lift. Research shows that happy people are motivated to do kind things for others, so therefore doing kind things will make you happier. Each day do one act of kindness beyond what you would normally do. These do not have to be over-the-top or time-intensive acts, but they should be something that really helps or impacts another person.

Some examples are the following:

- help a friend or colleague with something
- give a few dollars or some time to a cause you believe in
- say something kind to a stranger
- become a hospital visitor
- volunteer for a shift at the local op-shop
- write a thank-you note
- give blood.

At the end of each day, list your random act of kindness in a notebook or keep a running note on your phone. At the end of each week, reflect on the acts of kindness you have done that week and it will give your mood a distinct lift!

# 35. Breathe through your nose.

Mouth breathing from the upper chest triggers the sympathetic nervous system, thereby accelerating the heart rate and increasing blood pressure, as well as stimulating our fight or flight response —hence the link with anxiety symptoms.

In a ground-breaking study by Japanese researchers Masahiro Sano, Sayaka Sano and Toshinori Kato published in 2013 in the journal, *NeuroReport* (Kluwer), it was found that an increased oxygen load in the prefrontal cortex of the brain is caused by mouth breathing and has been shown to be a contributor to ADHD. (It was also found that mouth breathers were more susceptible to dry mouth, bad breath, the mouth hanging open, dental caries and gingivitis, snoring and smoking.)

In a further study by Japanese researchers Miho Nagaiwa, Kaori Gunjigake and Kazunori Yamaguchi at Kyushu Dental University in July 2015, it was found that it takes a longer amount of time to complete chewing to obtain higher masticatory (chewing) efficiency when breathing through the mouth. So, mouth breathing will decrease the masticatory efficiency.[28]

So, take action and stop breathing through your mouth. Here are some suggestions:

- Practise breathing through your nose and ask your family and friends to help you by pointing out when you are not doing this.
- Clear any nose blockage.

---

28 *Breath, The New Science of a Lost Art* is a fascinating book by James Nestor, available also as an audio book.

- Irrigate the nose by sniffing a salt-water solution up each nostril. Devices to assist this are obtainable at pharmacies.
- Reduce your stress by practising the techniques you have learnt.
- Use the correct pillows.
- Take regular exercise.
- See a therapist.
- Consider surgery if the cause is physical.

# 36. Count your blessings!

Gratitude is possibly the most important of all the above strategies because it brings happiness. *Count your blessings!* This old axiom makes us look at the positives in our lives and lifts the mood. Whenever we start to feel down, it's a good idea to use that four-letter word yet again, STOP!—and then list the things in your life for which you are grateful.

*Gratitude is so liberating—make gratitude a way of life.*

It's a good idea to keep a gratitude diary. Another good idea is to write to a friend and say how grateful you are to have them as a friend and the reasons why you feel that way.

Before you go to sleep each night, review the good things that happened that day and be grateful. A grateful person is one who accepts all of life (good and bad) as a gift. They see life as a gift and not as a burden. Grateful people are happier and do good things—they are generous, compassionate and forgiving.

Gratitude is an antidote to envy. Often a silver medallist on a podium is less happy than a bronze medallist. The silver medallist envies the gold, feeling he/she has fallen just short of the top award, while the bronze medallist is grateful just to have made it onto the podium.

# Conclusion

Anxiety and depression have now become pervasive. Drugs have for too long been regarded as the universal panacea. We have lost sight of the fact that we are resilient and resourceful human beings and that within us all is the power to shake off labels and regain control of our mental health simply by changing the way we think. Just four to six weeks of daily practice will bring about exciting positive change. I hope this guide has given you the confidence to connect with your amazing inner resources, change the way you think, and free yourself from the emotional virtual prison of the mind.

# References

Below are some links that you might find interesting.

Diet is believed to pay a big part in mental health.
Professor Felice Jacka from Deakin University is a leading
researcher in this field.
https://foodandmoodcentre.com.au

Dr Duncan Double: Relationships in mental health.
http://criticalpsychiatry.blogspot.com/

*The effect of social environment on mental health.*
Prof. Scott M. Monroe, University of Notre Dame.
https://psycnet.apa.org/record/2002-01778-013

Prof. Lucy Bowes: Oxford University interview.
https://www.youtube.com/watch?v=37gWY6tGW60

*The unfulfilled promise of antidepressant medication.*
Dr G. Davey and Dr A. Chanen in the Medical Journal of Australia
(May 2016).
https://onlinelibrary.wiley.com/doi/abs/10.5694/mja16.00194

Prof. David Healey: the over-prescription of drugs.
https://davidhealy.org/

*How do antidepressants trigger fear and anxiety?*
Dr Catherine A. Marcinkiewcz and Christopher M. Mazzone
University of North Carolina Medical School.
https://www.sciencedaily.com/releases/2016/08/160824135045.htm

*Working hours regulations and fatigue in transportation: A comparative analysis.*
Christopher B Jones and Drew Dawson
https://www.sciencedirect.com/science/article/abs/pii/S0925753505000299

Dr U. Wagner: Sleep study.
https://www.theguardian.com/science/2004/jan/22/research.science1

Depak Chopra: Guided sleep meditation.
https://www.youtube.com/watch?v=DxT9fTYgJcg

Eckhardt Tolle: Stillness meditation.
https://www.youtube.com/watch?v=fWEX3SRX7Ro

Sadhguru: Sleep meditation.
https://www.youtube.com/watch?v=Sm4ZBvDqD00

*A wandering mind is an unhappy mind.*
https://news.harvard.edu/gazette/story/2010/11/wandering-mind-not-a-happy-mind/

*Mindfulness practice leads to increases in regional brain grey matter density.*
Britta K. Hölzel et al
https://pubmed.ncbi.nlm.nih.gov/21071182/

Dr Bruce Lipton: The Biology of Belief.
https://youtu.be/PKEypjabGcA